MW00914865

The
OWNER'S MANUAL
To Living Your 40s
at Full Strength

12 Essential Life Hacks
for Your Best Decade Yet

SHAWN PHILLIPS

ISBN-10: 1494471272
ISBN-13: 978-1494471279

Welcome fellow Man...

Welcome to your fifth decade on this amazing planet. Congratulations to you on your successful journey, thus far. Trust me, it has been successful for you are here reading these words. Like all of us, I'm sure you've had a few detours, learned a few lessons and celebrated often. For all that has come before you are wiser. Now is your chance to apply that wisdom, to look forward with optimism, not back with regret.

It strikes me that at the tender age of 20 men have little to lose and the world to gain. Risk is called adventure. And at 40 these same men have everything to lose and risk is an enemy of security and we all begin playing a smaller game—aiming for singles rather than swinging for the fences. And of course there is some wisdom in this, but more often it's simply an unconscious shrinking of life, or reach, or courage. And it costs us all dearly.

As Helen Keller said, *"Life is a daring adventure or nothing at all."* It is my most sincere wish that your 40's be the best, most abundant, ecstatic and fulfilling decade of your life—and that this concentrated guide be the start of a new daring adventure that stretches you to the limits of your being, and well beyond. This is your day, this is your time, this is your life. Seize it now.

I'm also here to warn you that while your 40's can be the most rewarding decade of your life, it can just as easily be a siren; bringing you 10 grueling years that will make your soul ache for relief. The choice is yours. Which will it be?

What you are about to uncover in this guide is *stuff* the modest man will never consider and the great man will regret not recognizing sooner. These are the *questions*, the *answers*, the *how's* and *why's* that will help you craft **your** 40's into the brilliant decade it intends to be.

The 12 Most Essential Life Hacks are the very pearls of wisdom that I wish I had known at 40. Some are mistakes I have made, things I have overlooked, areas where I was ill-prepared. Others crafted from experience and reflection. Sure, I could have regret but I am also blessed by **a challenging 40's so you do not have to!**

My Big Swinging 30's

My 30's were an extraordinary ride at the top of life. Together with my brother Bill, and a lot of great, inspired people, I'd help to build the world's largest sports nutrition company, EAS; traveled the world, been part of my Denver Broncos' winning back-to-back Super Bowls, and was of the most well known physiques in fitness; to name a few highlights.

Even as 40 loomed on the horizon, I was sporting one of the most shredded, balanced, natural physiques in the world; had just released a best-selling book, _ABSolution_ and was living The Life: Single, a big house on the hill, with more German cars than I could count. I had the world by the balls. All was well... or so it seemed.

I had money, fame, and freedom and my 40's would be the decade to leverage it all, to soak it in and really live the dream. I dove into my 40's with naïve enthusiasm.

A few short months into my 40's I'd crashed my Harley off a steep, rocky canyon, barely escaping the worst of fates, welcomed my first child, a son, and was planning my wedding. Within the next 20 months, married with child, I'd lost a business due to an ugly partner conflict, my father had passed away suddenly, and I was just beginning to question everything I thought was true about life.

And that was just the beginning of the wild ride called my 40's which was determined to teach me, to challenge me beyond what I ever could have imagined. I learned about loss, about money, about opportunity, about love, about family, about pain and about presence. About waking up and really stepping into life from a ground of true strength, not ego or power.

If Only I'd Known

As I move ever closer to the end of my 40's, looking back at the wisdom I gained—mostly the hard way— these are the things I wish I'd known, then. These are the questions, the practices, the awakenings that had I taken them to heart, be proactive, had my eyes and ears open, would have made an enormous difference in the unfolding my decade.

I believe pain teaches us and challenge awakens, but let's face it, most of the shit that beats us awake is stuff we could have avoided had we known to "look out" in advance.

This is not a guide to making your 40's super-easy or stress-free, but rather to soaring through them gracefully and learning what you need with your eyes wide open. It's a bit of a road map—or a traveler's guide—to help you get the best out your 40's and enjoy the teachings rather than get them the hard way.

Maybe you will transform your marriage without losing it first. Maybe you will transform your wellness without getting ill first. Perhaps you can generate more wealth without losing it all first. There are so many ways you can make the best of what's to come and this short, simple, clear and crisp **Owners Manual** can be the most helpful, powerful change making guide you'll ever know.

- What you'll find in this book is the most concentrated, simple, lessons ... the "what I wish I knew."

- You'll come to know that while it *is* about your body—about health and wellness—it's more about the Strength of mind, heart and living a life worth remembering.

- How to love every day of your 40's, as if you'd chosen it with all your heart, even when you didn't.

The New Rules at 40

When I hit my 40's I recognized that there was a real problem for men in this phase of life. It's sort of the sandwich decade. You're not old enough to be somebody but you're too old to care about it. Other than Viagra and your pending AARP card, few seem to give a damn about you. There's little support and no guidance on how to be a better, brighter real man. I think you should know how *not* grow old—at least older than you have to—and how not to be stuck wearing kid's clothes or dressing like someone's dad.

Your forties are the first age you start to feel the sinking, the decline. Up until this point in your life, for the most part, the only change you've known is the growth kind; the good kind. The "getting better, stronger, more of everything."

As forty sets in, you begin, for the first time in your life to sense that there's a limit to what you can do. You know you've benched your best PR, you've reached your peak in so many areas. But you're good, your getting on... then, you realize that your energy is whacked. You can't keep up with endless hours and you can't go days without sleep. You're mortal after all—and that's not fun nor funny to feel.

Then, one day as you're feeling bad about your pending mortality, you eat a load of crap food and your body feels like it's trying to kill you. It doesn't just take it in and say, "thank you!" You literally feel like you've been poisoned, like you're sick as hell.

As I said in my best-selling book, *Strength for LIFE*, "age is less the result of the number of years you've lived than the way you've lived your years.," It's true that most men grow old before their time and then just when men have the most to offer the world they are losing their strength, energy and desire to share it.

It was this recognition of this "gap" that inspired me to create *Full Strength nutrition*. I knew that even *my* body was changing and that my life demanded something more, something different; a perfectly balanced, life enhancing, delicious performance meal rather than another "muscle building protein shake." Not that there's anything wrong with a protein shake, not for the 20 year old bodybuilder or athlete. But life changes and you must change with it or ahead of it.

Change is always better than the option. For the options are either you're dead or you're trying to resist change—a fine line there. These *12 Life Hacks* will have you embracing—even celebrating change—put you in control and help you live your 40's on top of life and fully in the game.

> *"Too often people let the decade define them, rather than defining the decade. Only through vision and intention can you bend life in your favor."*

The Magnifying Decade

Your 40's are the decade, where everything gets magnified. Have some health challenges that were nothing big but you've ignored them—welcome to your 40's where this becomes the dominant theme of your existence.

Have a little emotional tick, a sort of funny avoidance of challenge in your 20's that got difficult in your 30's—by your 40's this "tick" is now a full blown problem. It's a disorder, addiction, or emotional block that is set to derail your life.

Look, be it in health, finances, affairs and love, I've made a lot of mistakes, done a few things right and learned a shit load. Had I these fundamental, *basic rules for living your 40's at Full Strength*, I am absolutely certain that I'd have both avoided some set backs and celebrated many more successes.

That's why I am eager and honored to share my experience and pay whatever life wisdom you may receive, forward.

This ***MANual*** is my gift to every man out there on your 40th birthday. It's the best gift I could have imagined receiving—and at a time in life when most of the world is taking from us, I hope you enjoy receiving this from me and find my experience valuable in your journey.

May you enjoy a ***life of challenge, achievement, contribution and joy...***

Here's to Your 40's *at Full Strength!*

Shawn Phillips

Table of Contents

Introduction v

About The Unique Writing Style 14

Step 1: GET REAL 21

Step 2: GET SELFISH 29

Step 3: GET ENERGIZED 41

Step 4: GET STRONG 50

Step 5: GET GRATITUDE 68

Step 6: GET CURIOUS 73

Step 7: GET SIMPLE 81

Step 8: GET ZEN 88

Step 9: GET GAME 98

Step 10: GET BIG 104

Step 11: GET PURPOSE 114

Step 12: GET CONNECTED 122

STEP 13: BONUS 134

BIOS 141

I dedicate this **Owners MANual**—this guide to the journey—to every 40 year old man who refuses to "go quietly" and chooses to awaken the giant within. May this be the most brilliant, rewarding decade of your life, yet.

About The Unique Writing Style

The book you hold in your hands, ***The Owners MANual for Living Your 40's at Full Strength: The 12 Essential Life Hacks,*** is the product of an innovative, new way of creating wisdom-rich content that is fun, fast and engaging to consume—that means easy to read. It's done in the way we communicate, a conversation. In this case, the conversation is very intentionally and skillfully directed by a masterful "conductor" (Dean) for the subject matter expert and author—who in this case is me.

The result is an incredibly positive, empowering and fun way to get the information that can change your life.

In the pages ahead, you will see the names of myself, **Shawn** (Phillips), the expert guest and primary author, and **Dean** (Jackson) the host, preceding our commentary. In the process of creating this Owners Manual, Dean took over for me as host of my podcast, *The Kryptonite Report* ***(KryptoniteReport.com)***.

With that, we begin:

Shawn: I've got a special show today. This is your host, *Shawn Phillips*, and I'm taking a bit of a swing to the other side today. I've got a special guest host today, Mr. Dean Jackson of the *I Love Marketing* podcast and author of a million other projects. So I'm switching to the other side, and *I'm* going to be the guest, and Dean will interview me.

Dean is a brilliant business mind and a friend of mine for about 20 years. He and Joe Polish, another good friend of mine, host *I Love Marketing (Podcast: ILoveMarketing.com)*, which is actually the show that inspired the **Kryptonite Report.** If you're in business and you don't know *I Love Marketing*, be sure to check it out.

Dean: Thanks, Shawn. I am so excited about today. I'm thrilled to do this with you because we sat together for a few days a couple of months ago and talked about this idea: men really need an owner's manual for their 40s. Who better than you to write that **owner's manual** and share all of your great advice with people? So, I'm excited because I can't wait to hear what you have to say.

Shawn: I'm excited, too, and I really appreciate you getting me focused on this opportunity. I went down to spend a weekend with Dean to get my vision clear on my business, what I'm doing.

Dean asked me, "What are you most passionate about right now? What's the greatest possible impact you can make in this world?."

I said, "***I'm really about getting that 40-year-old guy back to the prime of life.***"

"All right," he said. "Let's do that."

And that's what I intend to do.

Setting your intention can be the simplest thing. It's always a good first move. Dean's inspired me to sit down and put this information together in a ***men's owner's manual*** for your 40s, including what follows, the 12 most fundamental strong moves.

Dean: I can't wait. We talked really getting clear on what the essential moves for your 40s. I think most begin to realize that the game has changed once you turn 40. I can't tell you how many times I've told the story you told me about the difference between your 30s and your 40s. You said that in you're 30s, when you'd get a headache, you'd pop some Advil and just keep going. In your 40s, you get a headache and you're scheduling a CAT scan to look for tumors.

That's so true!

Shawn: It is. When I wrote *Strength for Life*, the preface is all about the turning 40 event. I still have this story that got taken out of the book, but it was about I'm in great shape, I'm 39, 11 months and 29 days, I've got a handle on it, no big deal. I wake up 40 and you think the world had just tilted off its axis, right?

Dean: That's right.

Shawn: I'm like, "What the hell is this?" The thing about your 40s is, it can be a *death* sentence or a *life* sentence. What are you going to choose? How are you going to use this hallmark? It can be a negative for women, but it's an opportunity for men. You're not dead yet, by any means. So, it's a time to step into something. How do we use this opportunity in life to step up, to awaken, to recharge, to refocus, and use it as a **turning point**?

Dean: I'm fascinated by that whole approach.

You're really great at getting clear on what to do and what the right actions are. I love that you've got it down to the 12 best decisions that you can make going into your 40s.

Shawn: Dean, I took it from your piece. You asked me, "What's the minimum effective dose? What are you going to do?" From a physical perspective, I know how important the physical is because a lot of guys say, when they're 40, they're fine; 41-½ and they're fine; but 41 and 7 months, then all of a sudden they're like, "Man, I can't lose this weight," or "I can't do this," or "I can't do that," or "I thought this 40 thing was a myth. Then, suddenly, everything about my energy and everything else changes." Right?

Dean: That's it.

Shawn: So, there's a physical aspect, but I'm also smart enough to know this isn't just a physical thing, because if you change your body and transform yourself, you can look good in the mirror and still have a whole bunch of life conditions which are going to take your ass down.

Dean: It feels like, too, when you get in your 40s, you're just kind of gaining momentum intellectually, mentally, and inspirationally. Then your body, just when you've figured it out, you've figured out your direction, your body and your physicality starts to decline. It's a match-up with your intellectual capability.

Shawn: So true. Just as you're making strides the descent begins.

Dean: Right, exactly!

Shawn: That's one of the things that I wrote about in the first chapters of *Strength for Life*, what I call the "shape of your life." Your life goes up like the cross-section of a speed bump. It arcs up, bends over, and then heads down. Most people think that down is mid or late 40s, or something like that. Technically,

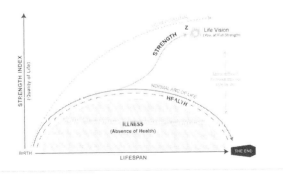

it's early 30s, but it doesn't really catch up with us until our 40s.

These guys in their 40s and 50s, who have the most to give back to life, have begun to lose their energy. If you lose your energy and can't give to the next generation or can't do your best music and play your best stuff, then the world loses. It's not just a personal crisis; it's a social crisis. You see people— exactly what you're talking about—losing it and not being able to get that *mojo* back and give their gift.

Dean: Yes, that's it. Tell me—let's go through our 12 here. I'm anxious to get some action steps going here.

Shawn: Yes, Dean, let's get down to the action— what should a guy do first? I say the first move of your 40s should be:

(For more info on Shawn and Dean, see their bio's in the last pages.)

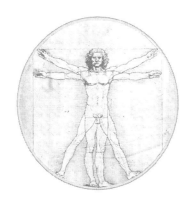

Step 1:
GET REAL

*Reality is the Domain of Strength
from Which All Results Arise*

Shawn: Get real man! I mean that as a kind of fundamental wake-up. Take a straight look in the mirror and get honest with yourself. This is the first step in any effective Transformation. If you look at *Body for Life*, one of the things Bill did is he had you take an inventory, confront the truth and "get real." That meant in part, taking your "before" pictures, and taking good hard look at where you're at, take your measurements, and know where you are.

Dean: I imagine you mean not just your physical measurements like your waist or those things, but really getting to know some of the key numbers that are going to be the most important, too. Is that what you're saying?

Shawn: Yes. I want you to physically know where you are, of course, but also where you are in every area of your life. In one of the groups I belong to, one of my forums, and we do an exercise every month to gauge our place in life—and being-ness. We've got this 7-sided "hexagon" that has a place for your health, body, mind; your business and career; your friendships; your financial; your level of giving; your spiritual ground; your marriage and relationships. On a scale of 1 to 10, you go around and rate each of those areas and determine where you are. You don't have to make it right or wrong, but simply evaluate where you are.

This is the part where you look at yourself, honestly assess, and grade yourself today, not where you have been, not where you're going to be, but where you are today. That honest assessment is the first step on a journey to figure out where you are, and decide how you're going to move from there. If we're lying to ourselves about where we are or we're keeping our head in the sand about it, we're not only going to miss a great opportunity, but we'll also end up off course.

Dean: Turning 40 is an ideal opportunity—although it feels like a momentous thing—to really take that self-assessment.

Shawn: It's definitely an opportunity. A door opens to a more awakened life, a more awakened radiance and passion for life. If you look at what it contributes to a transformation, an honest assessment is a catalyst for change. You really can move from a ground of strength when you're in integrity with where you are. If we're spending more than we're earning, we're pretending like things are better than they are, we've got our head in the sand about our physical well-being or our marriage or relationship, then we're setting ourselves up for a rough 10 years and beyond.

Dean: That's the thing, I guess, using it to make a decision. You can see where there are opportunities for improvement.

Shawn: That's it, and I think Jon Benson had a good one a while back. I believe he talked about the myth of balance, which is that we have this fantasy that everything in life is going to be balanced. Life's not always balanced, but things should trend towards better. There are areas where I'm never going to be a perfect "10" but that doesn't mean I should give up or just avoid placing any attention of focus on it.

Dean: At certain times, you do go out of balance intentionally on some things, but being aware that it's not going to continue and you're not going to let it slide forever.

Shawn: That's an awareness thing. At the end of all these steps I have a "Do This," list of only 1 to 3 things. The "Do This" on the 40s is just practice.

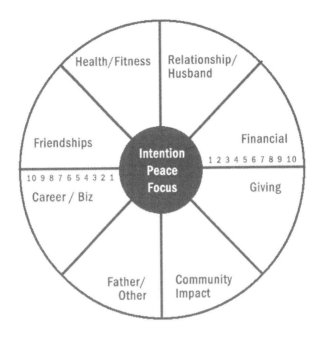

DO THIS:

Here is the chart I spoke of—this one is yours to go through it. You're going to take 10 minutes. You're going to look, assess, and say, "I'm turning 40 or ___. This is a great time for catalysts and to upgrade myself on these 7 areas. Where am I at?"

Now you've got your map. Here I am, in my 40s, examining where I'm at in my life and maybe even put a where you want to be on it. Where are you? I can tell you right now that the marriage and relationship isn't so hot, but it's an honest assessment.

Dean: Right. Awareness precedes momentum.

Shawn: And awareness is the gateway to freedom. You can't do anything with what you don't admit or don't know.

Dean: That sounds like an easy thing for somebody to do. I agree with you that concentrating your very best advice for guys entering their 40s is narrowing it down to these 12 steps. Number 1 is "**_Get Real_**," and here we are. We've got the chart for you to go ahead and do it.

Shawn: It's also a great time to look at where you're at physically in greater detail. You can take the entry stuff out of **_MyStrengthforLife.com_** book which, such as your stats, your measurements, where you're at, and so on. One of the things in _Strength for Life_ I ask people to do is keep an annual log. And every year, on their "best day of the year" when they have a physical peak, they should record their numbers; their weight, their well-being, their blood work, and record it to keep a running journal of their beingness. You'd be surprised at how fast 10 years go by and, all of a sudden, now you've got this history.

Visit: **MyStrengthforLIFE.com/Resources** to download this worksheet

Dean: Boy, it does fly. It just seems like yesterday that I turned 40.

Shawn: Don't talk to me, dude! I'm like, wow. I don't know whether to scream it out loud and be proud of it or walk around in humility. I'm not sure.

Dean: Just show them a picture of your abs. That's all.

Shawn: Yes, that's all.

Dean: You don't even need to lift up the shirt anymore, just show them the picture.

Shawn: I know. I look good. Every life has its ride and you have to be where you are. I think that's the fun in this. You said the word "concentrate." I think the value of what we're offering here in the owner's manual is a *concentrated* way to gauge, correct, invigorate, and inspire your life in a way that you can apply and do now. There are a lot of books out there, but they're also big, thick, and rich with all this to-do stuff, half of which you'll never even touch.

Dean: Right.

Shawn: These *12 steps are really tangible things* that you do in 10 or 15 minutes, and start doing right now. They're actionable steps.

Dean: I love it. So, number 1 is **Get Real**. What's next?

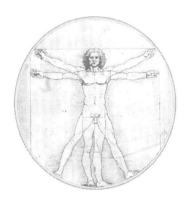

Step 2:

GET SELFISH

The Strength Begins with You

Shawn: I love selfish. Selfish, I think it sounds wrong, but it's completely right because men are so prone to the self-sacrifice. If often feels like I'm last in line behind my work, family, and everything else in the world. We sacrifice everything to try and provide and do the things that we're supposed to do. But there truly comes a point where putting yourself first *is* the **most** important gift you can give your children, your family, your career, because self-care is strength. It is the ground of strength. Be selfish with your time. You've reached your 40s. It's time to stop pissing your time away with everyone who wants you to do something for them.

Dean: When you say to get selfish, it reminds me of the instructions when you're on the airplane. If the air masks come down, secure your own mask first, and then help somebody you're with to secure their mask.

Shawn: That's perfect—the gold standard analogy. Secure your well-being first. I always loved that. Gary Vaynerchuk did a talk, I think it was *Web 2.0* or something about 3 or 4 years ago—when he just got up there and screamed to everybody in the crowd, *"Stop doing shit you hate."*

Dean: Right! But, you know what? One of the most famous things Steve Jobs is known for is his talk at Stanford where he said we should look in the mirror and ask, "If this is the last day of my life, am I thrilled about doing what I'm doing today?"

Shawn: Exactly. I think that's a question I can answer. I have days where I'm worn out, I'm struggling or something, but I always feel like I'm giving to a cause that matters and I'm committed to something. As we go through these steps, you'll find some of these are really about that kind of alignment.

One of the things—you see this throughout life— that comes up is how friends come and go. That's one of the things I've had issues with: people don't want to let go of certain friends. It's not that you're better than or worse than, but with some friends, it reaches a point where they're not bringing anything to your life. They're not on the same wavelength. They're not doing the same things you are, and you just have to move, not away from them, but just move on.

Dean: What is that saying? Something like people come into your life for a season, or a reason?

Shawn: Yes, exactly. It's simply ending that obligation, not doing things out of guilt, not sticking around just because you're good for them or something. It isn't selfish, but it's the most helpful thing you can do for everyone.

Dean: That's interesting. It's almost like pushing the **reset button** in a lot of ways, right? Like when you're moving into a new era here where you're living in a new decade. It makes sense to do that, coupled with an assessment of getting real, and then getting selfish and realizing what I'm sacrificing and what's stopping me from really working on what I now clearly see are things that need improvement.

Shawn: I think the reset button is the perfect analogy. That's what we're talking about. This point in life is a watershed moment, **a turning point**, an opportunity to recalibrate everything. What we do over the course of our lives is collect things. We collect obligations. We collect activities. We collect stuff.

Dean: It's like inertia then, isn't it? You just keep dragging it along, and now you're doing it because

that's what you've always done and this is who

you've always done it with.

Shawn: Yup. There are some great stories around that. It's like, "Why are you doing that?" "Well, it's because that's what I've always done." Right? That is the answer. It's just the way it is.

Dean: Do you know what's interesting? This really fits with what Dan Sullivan talks about, this idea of the immigrant mindset. You often hear tales of people immigrating from other countries, coming here with nothing, and then they, in a very short period of time, rebuild and exceed everything they had in their previous life.

There's nothing as freeing as being an immigrant. It's the ultimate reset button. They're completely removed from your environment and many times, they have nothing coming there. What they bring with them is their experience. Your brain comes with you. Your skills come with you. All of that stuff comes, but what you leave behind, even more important than the stuff, are all the commitments, the routines, and the relationships that were dragging you down or holding you back.

Shawn: That is a great analogy. As you said it, I got this sense of freedom and this idea that you can't drop everything in life, but so many things are simply about changing your environment, changing your habits, and resetting the stuff that's been unconsciously dragging you down.

Dean: Do you think that's why people come back sometimes so strongly from bankruptcies or from situations where they almost let go, and it creates this opportunity like the phoenix from the ashes?

Shawn: It really is. You hear the story over and over—whether it's bankruptcies, addictions, illness—ultimately, the freedom, I think, is through surrender. People think of surrender as a weak thing, as a collapse. **Surrender is a move of strength**.

I don't have that one in here, but the selfish has a piece of that in it of the surrender and letting go of it all so that you hold on to you. What you're really doing when you surrender to all the things you've been holding up or trying to hold up is you grab hold of the self. You take me away, and guess what, you can always build yourself back and all the stuff that was hurting or that you were holding or that you were juggling, it just hits the ground and you realize it wasn't that big a deal, but you were holding it all up.

Dean: So, how do you do that?

Shawn: Well, to do this is simple. Sit down, make yourself a "**Stop Doing**" list. This is a practice out of the Jim Collins' book, *Good to Great.* I always loved it's not the "Things to Do," it's the "Stop Doing" list. I look at the "Stop Doing" list as going on a 30-day commitment diet, which means you get rid of all the junk foods in your life for 30 days. Say, "Look, I'm going to eliminate every possible commitment for the next 30 days and see what kind of time crunch I'm really in. If I don't have to do it, I'm not going to do it."

Dean: You and I talk about this all the time. We're just full of ideas. There are so many things, so many opportunities, so many projects that we have kind of half-going that aren't completed. They're all great ideas. I've found it very useful, especially when I'm feeling like there are so many things going on, to make that list of things that I don't need to think about for the next 90 days. If you take all of those things—and I love this whole idea of doing a brain dump and getting them all out on paper—you'd be surprised that in 50 minutes you can get all of the things that are on your mind out there on to paper.

There's amazing freedom in looking at them and really assessing, "Will this still be a good idea 90 days from now? Does it need to be done right now?" There's such a sense of freedom when you acknowledge—you're not completely rejecting the ideas—but you're putting them on hold or moving them over here to clear some space for 30 days, 60 days, 90 days, just to really get selfish. I haven't thought about it like that, but that's really what it creates the space to do.

Note: "The 50 minute focus finder" is a Dean Jackson Process.

Shawn: That's an excellent practice, and I've heard you share that one before and I think I've done it a few times in my life. It's great, too, because you don't even have to make the decision on whether to kill it or not; you just make the space for now, **so push it out for 90 days**. That's awesome. **90 Days is key.**

Dean: Yes.

Shawn: I think that's definitely what we want to share, a kind of a commitment makeover.

One other thing I talk a lot about for guys especially is create some *sanctuary* in your life. Where is it that you have some space? It's a physical, an emotional, and a mental space. Where is your space of sanctuary? Where do you sit quietly and read? Where do you get some "me" time? Most guys, while being social or not as social as women, they need to sit on the big couch in front of the hotel or whatever it is, right? Where am I getting some time to just sit? Sanctuary is one of those words that has a real significant meaning. In the 1950s and 60s, men had a den or something.

Dean: Now it's called the "man cave."

Shawn: Yes. They called it a den because you growled in there, right?

Dean: Right.

Shawn: I watch *Mad Men*. I know how life was.

Dean: That's funny!

Shawn: I'm like, this is not all bad. The cigarettes are killing people, but it's not all bad. There are some aspects of that kind of life that might still work. I don't know. When you look at that now, it's like, I have an office at home and, god forbid, I go in there and I close the door because now I'm cutting off my family, I'm being anti-social and all these things. But how do I set physical, emotional, and healthy boundaries that support my *sanctuary*? Sometimes that can be in the gym, sometimes it can be on the bike, sometimes it doesn't have to be sitting. It has to be someplace that's my time and almost a recovery or regeneration "me" time.

Dean: I love that. Especially with how connected we are now with our iPhones always right at the end of our arm there, creating that sanctuary and that space is getting away from that. I joke sometimes that if I go play golf and don't take my phone with me, I say that I'm going to go golfing like it's 1989.

Shawn: Very Funny.

Dean: When there's no texting, no Facebook and Twitter, none of that stuff. The first time I did it, I felt naked, disconnecting like that. But also, I became really aware of how green the grass is, "Wow, look at all this stuff!" because I was looking up and taking it all in now.

Shawn: Wow, that's a really, really good point for sanctuary. It's a great example, and the golf course is a beautiful space for that. That's another good rule: disconnect. That's a great add-on—just disconnect. You feel vulnerable even at the thought of it, but then you get that freedom because we're never actually here if we're not taking it in. Physically, being here isn't the answer. That's the part of it. When I ride, other than there's some training I do with the *I Love Marketing* podcast in one ear, by and large, 90% of the time I am on the bike, focused on the bike, on my breathing, on my stats, on where I am, just being there.

Dean: I do that, too, but I've started going back and listening to podcasts and just keep feeding my mind at the same time.

Shawn: I appreciate that. I think it's a dual purpose, and it allows me to feel effective. I think that's part of why I brought Scott Tousignant on the (Kryptonite Report) show. I love Scott, but Scott and I do the **Kryptonite Report** together because I love how you and Joe have the play. It's a fun counterbalance, right?

Dean: Right. Exactly.

Shawn: It's a great one. The third one… ready for number 3?

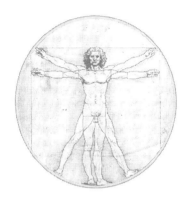

Step 3:

GET ENERGIZED

Energy is the Currency of Life
Time is for Clocks

"The Currency of Life is Energy." You can't get anywhere in your 40s, your 50s and beyond if you can't get energized, right? We are fooled into believing that all life is run by the clock, as if this is truly some Newtonian existence. Thus, we live, frantically, always in this time crunch when the reality is that energy is the currency of life.

Energy.

That is the currency of life. It's not time. We think it's time because we wear a watch, worship clocks, but all that we do is based on the amount of energy that we have to put into it. When your energy is high, you're focused and on, time is *your* servant. It does as you desire. When you're depleted, frantic, praying to the gods of hope and coffee, time can subordinate you.

Everything is energy—your willpower, your motivation, your stamina. It's all about energy now and sustainable energy.

So, you really must ask—or at least I must—What is energy?

Where does energy come from? One thing I've noticed and really dealt a lot with, I continue to feel more respect for the importance of energy as I get less youthful.

Dean: "...as I get less youthful!" What a great way to say that! "I'm getting less youthful."

Shawn: "Less youthful." I really think that *energy debt*™ is the true, great American crisis at this point. We are in an energy debt and our energy crisis isn't oil. Our energy crisis is physical, mental, emotional energy. Hence, we're addicted to caffeine. We've got all these stimulants. We've got all these things...

Dean: Artificially jumpstarted, right?

Shawn: Yes. Everything we do from checking our Facebook account to emailing someone, to exercising, to eating, to drinking our coffee and sugars, all the things we do are all **short-term stimulants** to pick us up, but they don't replenish our energy.

Ultimately, energy—there is such a huge component that is related to hormone balance, to lifestyle balance, to wellness, so there's a part of it that's energy, but there's really something when you turn 40 about embracing the vital nature **of rest and recovery**. That is, it's been proven that lack of sleep, pushing yourself to endless lengths, is going to kill you.

I remember in our 20s, we'd so boldly say, "I can sleep when I'm dead." If you say that in your 40s, you'll wish you were if you don't sleep.

Dean: That's so funny. I'll tell you, though, a few years ago, I really started getting serious about sleep and kind of studying sleep. I read a great book called **Super Sleep**. I don't know if you're familiar with it...

Shawn: I know the book.

Dean: I found *fascinating* the whole concept of sleeping in 90-minute cycles. I recognized it in my own life. Anybody who wakes up without an alarm clock, if you have that opportunity, you'll realize that if you take a look at when you go to sleep and when you naturally wake up, it will be invariably at a 90-minute increment. It could be 6 hours, it could be 7 ½ hours or whatever it is. I was intrigued by some of the stories in there of people who were chronically tired, but who went to bed at the same time and got up at the same time. It just happened that they were waking up in the middle of one of these 90-minute cycles and woke up completely groggy for the rest of the day.

The solution was having them stay up 45 minutes longer rather than go to bed earlier. They would wake up at 6 hours instead of waking up at 6 hours and 45 minutes or about 7 hours in the middle of a cycle. It made them so much more energized and productive throughout the day. The good news is, you can bank sleep, too. You can catch up. You can go with 6 hours for a few days, and then bank up with 9 hours one night.

Shawn: That's interesting because I'm a 6-hour sleeper. I'm not a 6-¼ , I'm not a 5-½… I know. I said it before that I can get away with 5-½ now and then, but it just kills me—6, I'm fine with. I can, once a week, do 7 or 7-½. But I'm a 6-hour sleeper and that's it. That's four 90-minute intervals.

Dean: That's exactly right. I'm totally into that. I think that Tempur-Pedic beds are the best. I love that sleep environment—the highest quality sheets, the right temperature… I keep the room at 66 degrees. It's just that I really got serious about my sleep and it made a big difference in my energy levels.

Shawn: It's vital. There is really only the vital energy, and that vital energy comes from the

regeneration of sleep. The absence of it, as you know—I heard you talk about it the other day—stimulates the production of cortisol, which drives our insulin, drives our weight gain, drives our disease, drives our body breakdown, it pushes down your testosterone, it suppresses everything. Stress will kill you. Stress is the same thing as the absence of sleep. They just go together.

Even though there are a lot of ways to get recovery and regeneration, all I'm saying is, you've got to take a new look at getting some respect and appreciation for the importance of recovery.

One of the things I teach in my book *Strength for Life*, is a mindful, Zen like strength-training practice. What I teach people when they're training with strength is that you've got 30 seconds to a minute of focused intensity training followed by a minute to 2 minutes of rest and recovery. People think that the training is the only thing that's doing anything. But you can only train as intensely as you can recover deeply. The space between the notes is what makes the notes.

"But you can only train as intensely as you can recover deeply. The space between the notes is what makes the notes."

Dean: Wow, that's interesting.

Shawn: The notes—it's the space, so you have to have space. You must have recovery between your sets. You need to have recovery between your days. You need recovery between your events. Even as much as a 50-minute work cycle, where you take a 10-minute break, a 15-minute or 10-minute break. That's helping you regenerate. That's helping you focus. That's helping you stay present.

My "Do This" on this one is really pretty simple. Once again, I suggest really taking a 12-day coffee break for people, and I'm a coffee guy.

Dean: Nothing but coffee for 12 days, is that correct?

Shawn: Yeah, yeah! Exactly! I want you drinking nothing but coffee, 6 cups a day for 12 days... That should be an interesting diet. How would that work? Hmm...

Take a break from coffee. The thing about coffee is you have to drink more and more and more of it to get less and less results. If you take a 12-day coffee break, you'll not only start experiencing what sleep should feel like, but the amount of coffee you drink when you go back—should you choose to return to drinking coffee, which most people do—will surprise you. You'll drink half a cup, and your hair's going to stand on end.

Dean: That's like turbo juice.

Shawn: Sure, like, "What the hell was in that?" You were drinking 3 cups 2 weeks ago, and you go back and have a half a cup, and you're heart's beating too hard.

Dean: Oh, I love it.

Shawn: But this is a reset. It's a great time to do a reset. It just helps you get a sense of sleep. Do what you were doing. Scheduling sleep as an A-list activity. Stop subordinating sleep to everything else you want to do from TV to books to reading to whatever. A nice little practice of quieting—this is one I've used off and on for years—doing 5 to 10 minutes of journaling before you go to bed to clear your head.

Dean: That's what I've started doing in the last 10 days. On my iPad, I have this Brushes app. During the last 10 minutes before I go to sleep, I make a little painting.

Shawn: Oh, cool.

Dean: Yes. The last 10 minutes of the day, it's just so relaxing.

Shawn: That's so cool. That's another great practice and another great way. I find that reading—because I like to read—that engages my brain is the wrong thing for me. So, if I start reading, I'll stay up all freaking night.

Dean: Right, because you get ideas and that starts stimulating things.

Shawn: Yes.

Dean: I was doing that same thing or doing something online or whatever, but this connecting with creativity part is turning that off. I find it relaxing. It's a little Zen thing.

Shawn: Totally. That's awesome. So, that was number 3.

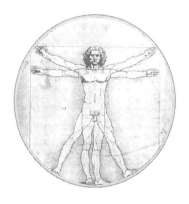

Step 4:

GET STRONG

Health is to Strength
as
Money is to Wealth

This one's one of my favorites. You know this one is me: **Step 4: "Get Strong."**

When I wrote *Strength for Life*, **Strength** was and is my entire meme—it's why I make *Full Strength Nutrition.* I really believe strength is not just a physical thing; it's a mental, emotional, spiritual aspect. It's about having more than just enough. When I looked at what health meant to people, if you look at health, health is defined consciously and subconsciously by most people as the absence of illness.

It's not the presence of anything. So, I say health is to strength as money is to wealth. Strength is an abundance of health. It is more than enough. It is having optimal health with abundant energy.

Dean: You know what's really interesting, because you and I have had that conversation before, the way that I thought about health was with upper and lower control limits. If you have strong at the top, sick or unhealthy at the bottom, and healthy in the middle, most people spend their life just trying to stay healthy. When they get sick, they only try to get back to healthy, where healthy is the highest level they reach. That really struck me when you were talking about strength. If you keep it in the upper half, if you're strong; if it slips back, you're just normally healthy.

Shawn: Exactly. It's moving the barometer. It's a new reset plan, a new standard. You're absolutely right that most people seek to maintain health. It's like seeking to maintain just enough money to not be bankrupt.

Dean: That's brilliant. I haven't thought about it like that. yes, just money and wealth. Being strong is wealth. That's something.

Shawn: It's not about a bench press or anything else. It's about treating yourself a certain way and thinking about yourself and working with yourself enough to build a capacity in reserve of abundance. It's an abundant life is what it is. As my Italian friend, Danny likes to say it's *Abbondanza!* That's "Abundance" in Italian.

Dean: Yes, that's it.

Shawn: Yes, abundance. I say when you look at people, it's like embracing your health as a gateway and a step toward the next level. It's about nourishing yourself and eliminating habits that are killing you and eating right instead. This is very much a physical aspect of it, and I'm a big believer in the importance of strength training because I know it's something that serves me very well.

As a guy, strength training has a unique capacity for changing your physical *beingness*. It doesn't merely change the way your body looks, but it also strengthens bones, strengthens muscle. Muscle changes the biochemistry, the chemistry of the body.

What we're learning and gaining more medical understanding of is that everything is about insulin mastery, when it comes to living leaner, longer and stronger. Insulin's your master control hormone and nothing can regulate, manage, and master insulin like more muscle tissue and strength training.

Dean: That's really fascinating.

Shawn: I stay lean with a good load of muscle. But when I eat a piece of chocolate cake, I start sweating because my body wants to utilize that...

Dean: And separate it.

Shawn: Yes, it starts burning it. "What are you

doing?" I say, "I'm burning off the cake." It's torching the cake at the moment because I have enough excess capacity to utilize this. Instead of my body saying, "Insulin, let's store this as fat immediately," it says, "Hey, pour that into the muscles because the muscles were cleansed of some level of energy through the strength training today." So, because of the muscles and the body-chemistry effects of strength training, my body can utilize it—and I have a wider margin of error.

Dean: A lot of times, guys coming into their 40s use this as a catalyst to lose weight, to get healthier, and focus on this. You and I have talked about the difference between burning fat versus building muscle. It was one of the most impactful things to me when you gave me an example. You took 2 identical people and one, over a period of time, did nothing but cardio and burned 10 pounds of fat compared to the other who did no cardio but gained 10 pounds of muscle. That 10 pounds of muscle they gained would go on and burn something like 40 more pounds of fat over a year.

Shawn: Exactly. It will burn the caloric equivalent of 40 pounds of fat.

Dean: Right.

Shawn: So you're striving to lose the 10 pounds of fat instead of gaining the 10 pounds of fat-burning muscle. I always like to look at it this way: if you can put 5 on and take 10 off, you've got a winning hand because the 5 on will help take the 10 off. We're not talking about you needing to pack on 40 pounds of muscle, because 10 pounds of muscle on a guy's body will change the way he looks completely.

It would be huge. That's a massive shift in the way you look and feel, and it strengthens the bones. The thing is, as we get less youthful, strength training becomes increasingly important as a vehicle for life. In the 10 greatest biomarkers of aging, all 10 are directly affected by strength training and dependent upon strength training. There's a huge scientific study looking at that. I like to say that strength training is just not optional. You don't have to go out and squat or deadlift the world. Simply use resistance to strengthen. There's a part of that, too, which fits in the psyche, the confidence, the power. I was just watching a **TED Talk** with, I think it's Amy Cuddy, who was talking about body language. She talked about how certain stances, physical stances, radically alter the **testosterone levels in men.**

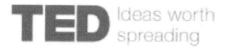

See **Amy Cuddy: 'Your body language shapes who you are'** on YouTube

Strength training is the most effective way of slowing down and even reversing the process of aging. In their book ***Biomarkers***, William J. Evans and Irwin H. Rosenburg covered 10 biomarkers, key physiological measures of the aging process. All 10, the authors said, could be favorably altered through strength training alone.

The 10 biomarkers are: *muscle mass, strength, basal metabolic rate, body fat percentage, aerobic capacity, blood sugar tolerance, cholesterol, blood pressure, bone density, and the ability to regulate body temperature.* The authors believe, as I do, that muscle mass and strength are the two most significant variables determining the quality of your life.

Dean: Really?

Shawn: A warrior stance or a strong stance or taking a position like a football player alters your testosterone levels.

Dean: That's interesting.

Shawn: I mean, that's more than just a stance. That's a physical expression to the world that gives you a sense of power. On my "Do This" list, I say it's not enough to exercise, you've got to **pick up heavy things.**

Dean: If you've got enough weight to lose, maybe you are the heavy enough thing.

Shawn: It doesn't matter, honestly. It's like body weight training is all the rage these days. Do whatever it takes. I put this one in here because every guy, as soon as they can in their 40s, needs to go get their blood work done. It coincides with your strength. You need to have a baseline mark. I want you to know what your blood work is. I want you to mark it. I want you to know what your testosterone and hormone levels are as a man because we're in a crisis these days. I think there's both an increasing awareness and a decreasing testosterone level across the board in men everywhere. If you don't know it—I mean, the suffering and silence for years at not being able to alter and change your muscle level tissues, being low energy... I always like to say, "How do you know if you've got low T? You're depressed, but you're too depressed to give a damn about it."

Dean: Oh, that's funny.

Shawn: You're almost comfortably numb. It's like, "Yeah, I don't know, maybe I'm depressed. I haven't really thought about it."

Dean: Oh, man. Take 10 guys, let's say, coming into their 40s. Is it that common that they're going to have low testosterone? Or is it genetic, or what's going on there?

Shawn: There are a number of things. There are environmental factors which include the estrogen mimickers like the BPAs (found in many plastics), the pollutants and contaminants in food and water that are affecting us. There's something a lot more than that. About 65–75% of guys are going to have some compromised testosterone levels. That's too many. It's too many just to be an accident. When I look at it, I look at the *lifestyle* factors, which are too much stress, too much alcohol, too much sugar, not enough sleep, too much cortisol, not enough good sex, not enough intense strength training, insulin levels all over the place. All these things contribute—5% here, 10% there. A scientific study was able to show that 50 grams of sugar lowered testosterone levels by 25% for 6 hours. Now that's frightening!

Note: A proven effective way to **kick-start your Testosterone,** naturally, is with a lifestyle change. By eliminating all the foods—junk and other—that spike insulin, cutting your stress level are reduced and your body can begin to regenerate and return to the optimal hormone levels it desires. The *12-Day ReBOOT* the first move towards fitness from my book, *Strength for LIFE*, helps you do just that. Simple, effective, proven the **12-Day ReBOOT** is like pressing the "ReBOOT" button on your body for renewed energy, clarity and Strength.

Visit: **fullstrength.com/12-day-reboot**

A Note About ED's

ED's are a Big Deal in this downward trend of Testosterone for men. ED, not as in the erectile dysfunction but as in ***Endocrine Disruptors***. One of the most well known is BPA, the stuff that was found to be leaching out of plastics and into our bodies. There well over 800 documented ED's in the environment that are actively impacting you and all men. They are in pesticides, food, water—in your foods and in the all the stuff your body is exposed to including soaps, detergents, dryer sheets and all manner of things that "smell" good.

It's not like you can carry a list around of ED's and keep your eyes open. The best way to avoid these ED's is to be aware of the major categories of products and begin getting them out of our life. Cleaning your fruits and veggies, well; eating organic, going hormone free; and ridding your environment of all the "smell good" stuff that contain them like soaps, detergents and avoiding room air fresheners, etc.

Dean: I remember you telling me that. That's fascinating. Just cutting out sugar, does it work? What's the corollary of that? Does your testosterone vary that much during the day?

Shawn: I think it is dependent on the day, but it's also what you do every day. It's the repeating, the repeating, and the repeating. If you strength train X number of days a week, if you get your sleep and you do the activities that support, it's not that you're trying to build this super hormone level; it's that you're trying to get back to optimal levels.

One thing I have a problem with about the urgency for treatment is that a lot of guys have artificially suppressed testosterone levels. It means that they've got a **lifestyle component**: they're doing 8 or 9 things that are suppressing their testosterone levels a little bit, which adds up to a lot collectively. Then they go in and they get treated, but they're treating the symptom, not the cause. The cause is their lifestyle's broken. If you don't make a shift in the way you live, you're going to over-treat, over-medicate, you're going to get more side effects, and you're still going to have problems downstream because you can't inject enough testosterone to solve a lifestyle problem that you're not treating.

Dean: I know a lot of guys, and this has become more and more common. Maybe the prevailing attitude is, "I can just get some shots. No problem. I can get my testosterone right back up." But it's like continuing to patch a roof that you haven't fixed the leak on, right?

Shawn: Yes. We're just bailing with the bucket, and this boat's still leaking. You know me, Dean, I'm a huge proponent of men's testosterone. I have been for 20 years. I believe that men really need to care for this number and know their number. I want men to "know your T" and get a hormone test, which hormone tests to get, how to look at a male hormone panel, what to ask your doctor for. I tell a lot of guys how to go to their doctor, how to ask for what they're getting, how to know if their doctor is going to help them or not. But I still say that you've got to look at a corrective lifestyle as a part of this either before or after doing it. That's why nutrition is a huge component about this, because if you maintain insulin levels, your blood sugar level stable and steady, that's a huge part because insulin is the enemy of testosterone and growth hormone.

Dean: It's really fascinating when you think about that. Just changing some of the lifestyle things, you've got access to 25% more testosterone. You were saying about not many grams of sugar affecting you for 6 hours. If you're eating that 2 or 3 times a day, effectively, your entire 16 or 18 hours you're awake, you've got 25% less testosterone than you have access to naturally.

Shawn: Absolutely. One of the great examples of how this can change is, a few years back I did that study at the **University of Oklahoma** on the ***Full Strength*** nutrition shake. We put about 80 people on *Full Strength*, they just added the Full Strength shake daily. They did a minimal amount of exercise—the same as for the exercise-only control group. There was another control group as well.

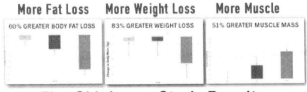

The Oklahoma Study Results

The participants who enjoyed the *Full Strength* daily, did so with zero dietary restrictions; they didn't have to change anything else they ate, they just enjoyed a Full Strength shake.

The results were **truly stunning**. This is the only study in the history of mankind (in the absence of anabolic hormones) that produced significant increases in lean muscle mass, while simultaneously losing body fat. What makes that so unique is that you lose fat in a calorie-restricted diet and you gain muscle with calorie-abundance. They don't happen in the same environment. They're polar opposites. But it did happen here. The *Full Strength group* added muscle, lost fat, dropped weight and even gained considerable energy.

Hence the reason why it took us 9 months to get this study published in the *Journal of Nutrition and Metabolism* because, as they asked, *"How could a nutrition shake have a drug-like result?"* The only way you see these things happen is if you change your hormones.

So, after many months of investigation, we finally concluded that the blood sugar-and insulin-regulating capacity of *Full Strength*—its ability to help sustain stable blood sugar throughout the day, what I call "insulin momentum"—had so altered the body's reaction of insulin, that it affected the way the subjects ate all day. It positively influenced the way people nourished their bodies and as a result, their bodies seemed to respond consistent with a more optimal hormone level.

Get a Free Full Strength 2-Pak Sample here:
http://FreeStrengthShake.com

It was amazing to see the researchers' faces and how startled they were when they saw this. "This could be the end of dieting." That's what the lead researcher said.

Dean: Wow.

Shawn: I have that on camera. He goes, "This could be the end of dieting." It just changed the way these people's bodies responded without *any* dietary restrictions.

That's the nature of getting your hormones under control. That's really what's behind a lot of the paleo-diet stuff. It's really about getting refined sugars, carbs, and things that are causing hyper-insulin responses out of your life, and allowing your system, your pancreas, and everything else to stabilize and level.

Dean: That's *fantastic.*

Shawn: So, the last thing that I will say on the "Do This" point is, I'm asking people to engage in a structured, training intensive program. Whether they enter some sort of challenge, whether they start some 12 weeks or 90 days of *CrossFit*, whatever you do, get a trainer, do something and make a commitment to do **a 90-day deep dive into strength**, into getting stronger, building muscle. Because once you get through the phase of understanding and creating a relationship with strength (and strength training) it will be a practice for life. It's like learning golf. You don't love the part where you're whacking the balls all over the place.

I'll tell you, I didn't love cycling for the first 90 or 180 days. Then I had to create a new relationship with my body, with a practice. And now I'll ride for life.

Dean: I love that. Okay, so "Get Strong." These are the "Do This" for "**Get Strong**."

DO THIS

- Pick heavy things up.
- Get your **T**estosterone tested.
- Engage in a structured training program for 90 days (*Strength for LIFE*, *Body for LIFE*, ***P90x***, what have you...)

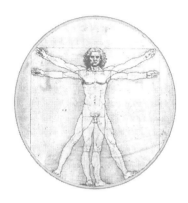

Step 5:

GET GRATITUDE

Training is to Fitness

as

Gratitude is to Happiness

Step 5: "Get Gratitude." Get a lot of gratitude, man. Gratitude is the muscle that cultivates happiness. I think we talked a lot about happiness. Happiness is a side effect. It's not a primary effect. You think, "Oh, you get happy." That's a concept of the mind; you don't make yourself happy. Really indulge in gratitude, and it's everywhere these days. The gratitude economy, we talk a lot about it. People have gotten much more popular with the idea of gratitude. I see cranky seniors who never developed the muscle of gratitude at an earlier age. That doesn't look like fun to me.

Dean: No. Exactly. That's an interesting concept. I haven't thought about that, that gratitude precedes happiness.

Shawn: That's the way I see it. Happiness as a mind concept. You don't force it, but if you're finding the gratitude in the moments, it comes to you. I'm an older parent with young kids—my daughter is 5 right now, my son is 9—I've cultivated the ability to be present. Every morning, it's the really Zen moments where I just feel incredibly blessed to be observing this life. It's my exercising of gratitude. It's my space.

I do bring a lot of gratitude practice in my strength training practices. We should be grateful for our ability to move and exercise our bodies. I mean, golf has got a lot of gratitude in it, man—I'm grateful that I hit a decent shot. And the thing about gratitude is gratitude begets gratitude. Some brings more… and more.

Dean: Every now and then, right.

Shawn: My "Do This" on this is pretty quick, down and dirty. There's a great video from the father of **Positive Psychology**, Dr. Seligman, and he has this thing called the "gratitude visit." He did it on a **TED Talk**, and I posted it on my StartStrongMonday.com blog, but I'll share the TED talk here. It's a short piece, about 10 minutes, where he talks about how to set up a gratitude visit with someone who has affected your life. It's a beautiful thing, and it's a great transformative thing. He talks about how deeply it can transform your experience of gratitude and other people.

Here's a great gratitude practice that I picked up somewhere. I call it the "14-day gratitude practice." For 14 days, put 3 quarters in your right pocket when you leave the house in the morning. During the day, every time you express gratitude or have a gratitude moment, take a quarter and put it into your left pocket. Try to go home at the end of the day with all the quarters in your left pocket.

Dean: That's fantastic—making that conscious because they're jingling around in your pocket.

Shawn: You'll start to pay attention and say, "I've got 3 gratitude moments today at some point. I might express gratitude to my office manager for something. I might have a gratitude moment online. I might go to Facebook." Whatever it is, take a moment and really reflect on it. I like a morning gratitude journal. Whatever it is.

These are just small practices that you can put in play today. I'm not asking you to do every one forever. This *14-day gratitude practice* is a great way to ingrain and start to feel the effects. You get to choose how this goes on in your life.

Dean: I like that. That's something that anybody can do. It doesn't really take any extra time. It's just a different awareness.

Shawn: Yes. I like having anchors. The quarters in your pocket are a terrific way for you to remember at the end of the day. Then you feel that sense of accomplishment. You go home at the end of the day or you go to close your day and you're like, "Oh, I did my thing. I did my thing." Repeating this exercise daily will strengthen your habits, strengthen your rituals.

Now, I'm ready for number 6.

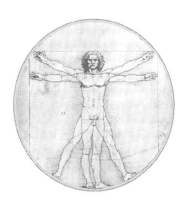

Step 6:

GET CURIOUS

*Because You Don't Know
What You Don't Know*

Alright, this one is my favorite, actually. It's really simple. **Step 6: "Get Curious."**

Dean: I love that. —I wanted to jump ahead because you—said, "I don't know where I pick all these things up."

I said, "I know exactly where you pick it up because you're curious."

Shawn: I think you really see this—it's an accidental decaying and apathy of the mind that we lose our curiosity. I find myself in a constant state of wonderment like a child. It's my ADD thing or whatever it is. I find something new or cool over the weekend about Bo Jackson that I didn't know and I think is really cool, or some odd thing that I pick up, or I listen to <u>Mary Ellen Tribby and *I Love Marketing*</u>, and I start sharing 4 things with people that I picked up.

Curiosity is an open mind. In the Buddhist view, they call it the "beginner's mind." Beginner's mind— to always have the mind of the beginner is to be enlightened, to be awakened. So often, when we know, I call it the "disease of knowing."

Because "I know" is the default stance for most adults. "I know" means nothing else is coming in, we are closed. This subject is dead to me.

Damn thing is you don't know that you don't know. So your mind thinks what it knows is everything. That's it's delusion. When you fall into its trap a part of you begins to die. Your mind stiffens, literally. You cut off openness, learning, opportunity and experience.

The way to opening isn't through "thinking" more though. It's through experience. If you think about something that you don't know, you by default compare it to something you do know. And that becomes your marker. Only through new experience do we really reshape and redefine what we know.

Dean: I would say that curiosity is what led me to studying sleep like that. There's such a big payoff for getting curious.

Shawn: I think it's ultimately *youthifying*, right?

Dean. It's *youthifying*! You know, curiosity is like the mental equivalent of a fresh sheet of paper.

Shawn: Exactly! And that's the beginner's mind, the blank slate. We're going to clean it up. We're going to go after something. I love the curious mind. One of the places we lose curiosity is in our closest relationships. My wife brings that up often, which is really embracing that curiosity, really being curious about the people around us in life.

That's why I have the "Do This" practice here. This is one of the things that you can do for 14 days, very consciously, and which will alter the way you're affecting your relationships with others. You might even see and experience the way it changed.

DO THIS

Ask 3 questions in your conversations with others before you share one thing. When your going to go see someone or meet someone, instead of thinking what you're going to share, start thinking, *"What am I going to ask Dean? What would be curious? I'm curious about Dean's—I'm curious about whether he's going to Necker Island this year. I'm curious about what's going on here."*

When you stop thinking about what your going to project and open your mind to what I'm going to be—

curious—then you've become mindful. That's what curiosity is: **mindfulness**.

Dean: That is interesting. I love how all these are kind of tying together, too, because I think if we go back to number 1 and get real, and we start looking at all of the areas that you were talking about—your health, business, career, friendships, financial, giving and contribution, spiritual grounding, marriage and relationships—then really applying curiosity to each of those, you ask, what can I get curious about in that realm?

Shawn: That's a great point. They unfold and then they fold back on each other for application. Certainly, *getting real (1)* is a foundation for creating some space for curiosity—*getting selfish (2)*, creating some space for **curiosity**, creating some space for **gratitude**. When I'm grateful, I'm more open to receive. There is this cascading aspect of these practices. I've shared a little bit about one of my few television obsessions and things I'm fascinated with, but like you, I love *How Stuff is Made*. Nathaniel, my son, and I, we just watch the hell out of that.

Dean: I think it's meditative. I go through this trance of watching all these processes. It's so good.

Shawn: I can't wait to figure out how they did the socks, man, like, "Check out that sock machine." It's so cool. How do they do that? "Oh, look at that!" The wife thinks we're nuts. But, I'm like, "Oh, that's cool." Did you ever see *Sliced*?

Dean: No.

Shawn: Oh, *Sliced* was so cool, man. *Sliced* was a guy—he played a commercial, kind of crazy, really good character. He'd take a giant saw and just slice things down the middle.

Dean: I have a friend who does that as a company—that's what they do. They make cutaways, that's what it's called. They take motors or any kind of product that you want to show the layers of, they'll cut it like you see in those trade shows and that kind of thing.

Shawn: Yes, he cut a fire engine in half one time.

Dean: Love it.

Shawn: Cut an armored car in half, but then he also cut an Etch-a-Sketch in half.

Dean: No kidding?

Shawn: He cut a garbage disposal in half to show you how a garbage disposal works. How cool is that?

A pinball machine. Anyway, we love that show, too.

I'm also really into *Mad Men* because I find myself curious about what was it like to live during that time.

Dean: Right. I think people feel the same about *Downton Abbey*. It's the same thing. It's curiosity—what was it like to be rich back then?

Shawn: It's another form of curiosity to put yourself in the shoes or the position of another person and have that experience of another time.

Dean: Curiosity almost feels like a luxury item. I think when you talked about creating the space for all these things, getting selfish creates the space for you to get curious. When you have the space and energy, one of the nice things to spend that on is curiosity.

Shawn: I like it as a luxury item—but an essential one. It's like rest and recovery. If you're always on and driven, and you're compulsively driven from a current state of fear or lack, then you're going to be sacrificing rest and sacrificing curiosity.

At some level, curiosity is also a part of your awakening and revival, so you're feeding yourself.

So, it's output and input. You've got to balance them.

That leads us to another fundamental one which is **Step 7: "Get Simple."**

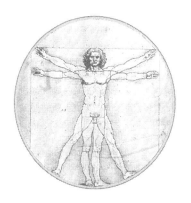

Step 7:

GET SIMPLE

*Because Less is More
and
The Best Beats The Most*

We hear a lot about simplifying these days, but in your 40s, you've got to look at the difference between stuff and substance; because we have collected all this stuff. We've got all this stuff. My garage is full of stuff. I don't know what to do with this stuff, but I don't necessarily want this stuff. I can't tell you, over the last few years, the amount of clothes that I have eradicated from my life. I used to be a clothes whore, right?

Dean: Used to be?

Shawn: Yeah. I still like clothes, but I just don't have the same condition and it's okay. When I got married and started sharing my house—I have a relatively large home—I had a walk-in closet in the upstairs hallway and 2 other bedroom walk-in closets all full of my clothes.

Dean: Great, great. I love that!

Shawn: There were at least a hundred pairs of shoes.

Dean: Why wouldn't there be?

Shawn: Sure, why wouldn't there be? Now, I have 8 pairs of chucks.

Dean: There you go. I love that. My favorites.

Shawn: Yes, you've got to love them. Simplifying, and part of simplifying, I think, is simplifying not just the stuff in your life, but getting back into the substance and things that fuel you. One of the things I talked about in my book *Strength for Life* is the difference between ***habits and rituals***. I love the *7 Habits of Highly Effective People*. It's a great use for the term "habits," but I think, largely, habits are things that we want to get rid of. "I have a habit of *blank*."

Dean: Oh, that's interesting—weaning yourself of habits.

Shawn: Yes, habits.

Dean: But you're using it in the positive way.

Shawn: I say rituals are life-sustaining, life-supporting things that we do ritualistically. It's kind of a holistic, well-being aspect to it.

Dean: Let's face it, we do the same things, eat the same things... We're quite comfortable with the habits that we currently have.

Shawn: Yes. I think it's nurturing those habits or rituals, the positive rituals that are supporting your life. One of the things that I'm big on is "repeat performances," nutritionally. Every meal doesn't have to be a unique work of art. I do some of the same things every day because they're hallmarks of excellence, gold-standard practices that I don't have to think about. I rarely have to ask, "What am I going to have for breakfast today? Let me contemplate that for 20 minutes." No. I awake, train and enjoy my **_Full Strength nutrition shake_**. It's complex nutrition that is a huge part of simplifying my life. It's the simple moves in life that create the space—yes, for rest, recovery, curiosity.

Dean: I think you've known me long enough, Shawn. I wear the same exact thing every single day. My black t-shirt, my khaki shorts, the black hat. The great simplification here is that it allows my assistant to pack for me without any kind of instruction. "How many days are you going?" Then it's this many shirts and that many shorts and that many underwear. There are no decisions or coordinating of what outfit am I going to wear when. It really has been such an incredible simplifier in my life.

Shawn: Think about how much **freedom** that creates. Just think about it. I do the same thing, too. I go to the office, but I work really just with me and my small team. I've been in that thing, too, where I'm big on the black t-shirts, I've got the black chucks or the flip-flop chucks or flip-flops on, and I go in the same every day, all the time, and just repeat it. It's refreshing. It's simplifying. It's part of keeping things simple.

I'm an every morning nutrition shake guy. That's my thing. I have been for 20 years. I don't have to get up in the morning and go, "Oh gee. How should I do my eggs today?"

Dean: Right, or "Should I have eggs today?" You're so right. That's really the brilliance of Full Strength: being able to get that part, that one thing a day, handled where it's just a part of the day and you don't even have to think about it.

Shawn: That's it. If you have your bedrocks that support and sustain your freedom in other areas, it moves a few decisions a day out of the way. It begins to create space and freedom because once again, let's go back. We don't know how much stuff has eaten away at our time, mental space, and freedom. So,

85

we're getting into our 40s, we've just turned 40, or we're entering this next turning point in life. Let's create the new freedom, the new space.

So, my **"Do This"** on *"Get Simple"* is—and this is one we probably need to do annually—but get rid of clothes you don't wear. What a clean closet looks like when you've got rid of the jeans that just are goofy and don't work anymore, and all this stuff that you don't need. Clean out your office and get rid of all the papers that you don't need. I went through and threw out all the back taxes that were years behind. I don't need them. They're done. All this stuff in America is in storage, limit everything you've got in storage. Just sell it. Sell it if you need to, but get rid of it.

Dean: Let them auction it off in *Storage Wars*.

Shawn: Yeah! Create some freedom in your life. This one is really important for me to start working on right now, but which I haven't done is, get rid of the books that I won't read again. Pass them on. Give them to other people. I have thousands of books, and I know when I see them on the shelf, I say, "I'm not going to read that again."

Then, what do I have left? Now I can walk into my library and find the books that I really do want to read again. The ones that are dog-eared.

Dean: You have them on your Kindle or your iPad now, too. It's amazing when you find your bookshelves full of thousands of books. That's something. The thinking is that, "I have every one of those books on one device," on your Kindle.

Shawn: I know. It's kind of wild. I'm a freak for physical books too, though. I just like the process, the feel of them.

The last thing on the "Get Simple" is how we need to apply it to your life. I say, we look at this life—we've talked about it before—it's a collecting endeavor. We're collecting; all this stuff is sticking to us. If we can throw some of this stuff overboard and lighten our load for the next act in life, it's so refreshing.

I've got friends that have gone through bankruptcy and lost everything. I mean, the brightness in their eyes and the joy in their step when they really get a taste of what it's like to have a simple life. I'm like, "Yeah, it looks like a pretty good idea."

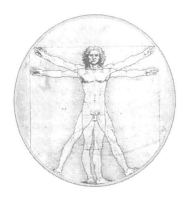

Step 8:

GET ZEN

End Your Wrestling Match
With Reality Now

It sounds cool, because it's in, it's vogue. But when I say "Zen," I'm referring to a life practice of getting free from all these things that we're attached to.

This follows "Get Simple" quite perfectly as this one is about releasing the stuff "inside" your mind. It's a state of *being*. We get attached to our ego, and ego is always battling for something to be different than what it is.

We want it warmer when it's colder, we want it colder when it's hotter. We wish we had less. We want more time. We're in a wrestling match with reality. That's eating our energy up and it eats us up. Getting free to me is really not so much as breaking things off, but getting back to that center and that ground.

One of the areas I look at when I talk about freedom as a real, tangible area is getting free from this idea of dieting. **Dieting** is what I call a struggle to control the way you eat. We're in this battle with our mind and our body, and it's this ongoing chess match. Instead of dieting, if you create what I call *Nutritional Freedom™* practice," where you reinforce a positive relationship with food, such that you'll actually choose to eat the foods that are best for you because they're the ones you desire most. That's freedom—to eat the food you really want that is also the best for you, and you're doing it effortlessly and freely—not in this restricted battle of dieting.

One of life's certainties is that quirks you pick up in your late teens or early 20s turn into full blown "issues" by your 40s. If you're talking full blown disorder, think Elaine—on *Seinfeld*. Elaine and Jerry are talking, "You're just a hop, skip and a jump away from a full blown disorder."

Those things that were cute or funny aren't cute nor funny anymore. They turn into addictions, compulsions, pathologies of some sort. This is the time that, if we're going to move on in life, we must start reaching freedom from these things that are driving us—by waking up.

We're not driving them, they're driving us. There are things I'm turning away from, things that I'm hiding from myself, things like the constant craving for more money; I can never have enough. We know how "never have enough" will work out for you: you'll never have enough. There's no satisfaction in it.

Dean: I said that to Tony Robbins about the story of the man who doesn't want to own all the land, just the land that's next to his. There's no end to that.

Shawn: Yes, exactly.

The Zen thing is a cultural movement these days. We like to talk about it. I'm not saying you have to move to some religious or spiritual practice and all, but I mean, we're talking more about being in a more centered, present state of mind. It's about dropping our illusions and getting really reoriented with our reality. If we can be with what "is," effortlessly, we're starting to lose that attachment. Attachment and our ego is really what starts driving us nuts. We all know people who are way too attached to their ego.

By gaining presence and getting into the awareness and being in the now, it's like Eckhart Tolle talks a lot about in *The Power of Now*. You can read or listen to *The Power of Now* a hundred times and it's hard to argue the truth in it. It's like there is no power in the past, and there is no power in the future. There is just now.

If we can get the present to what is now, deal with what is, that's the origin of all freedom, and from that, what infinite curiosity, what infinite energy… What do we gain? We just released this tornado of struggle that we've had in ourselves. I'm not saying that it's the easiest thing in the world to do, but it is certainly doable.

Dean: I'm thinking about this and looking at my notes on this, the yin and the yang, the back and forth of what's happening here. *Get Real. Get Selfish. Get Energized. Get Strong. Get Gratitude. Get Simple. Get Zen.* Simply bringing an awareness to this collection of things is pretty powerful, just looking at my notes here.

Shawn: Well, it's cool when I hear it because you can feel the energy in the yin-yang of it. The yin-yang, the polarity is what drives all action and movement in life anyway. Any one of them kills off both of them. That's the real balancing act. That leads us to the practices that do this.

One of the practices in the "Get Zen" is—I'm going to share the practice from _Strength For Life_ that I call the **Nutritional Freedom**™ practice." It's a **mindful** eating practice. It's got a beautiful diagram and graph that show you the change in relationship from the time you get hungry to the time you quiet your hunger. That's how we relate to food. Its function is to quiet that "crazy Aunt" in my tummy that gets starving and to make it go away. Then we get sleepy, slobber on the desk, fall, and pass out, and then we don't know why we did that because we don't have any relationship to the cause or effect or the back end of how food obsessing makes us feel.

When I show you how to change your awareness,

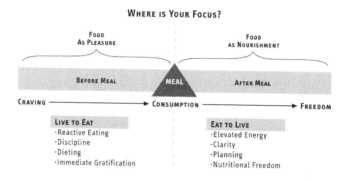

WHERE IS YOUR FOCUS?

to shift from the front end to the back end, so that you relate to food from how it feels from the time you eat it to 1, 2, and 3 hours later, the freedom begins. Now you've created a feedback loop, and you go, "Well, that really tanked me," or "That really picked me up." You start to create a positive feedback loop, and that's self-reinforcing.

Suddenly, you'll be eating well, effortlessly.

93

Dean: They don't think about how it's affecting them.

Shawn: The graphs, the visuals, and the little practices are really great. Like Dan Sullivan, I like to draw visuals and diagrams to help you see what I'm getting at. This is one of the really strong fundamentals in this book *Strength For Life* that I want to share here, because this is how you rewire your future food and nutritional consumption.

If you practice Nutritional Freedom you will begin to realize that the primary function of food is to fuel your wellness, strength, and energy. When you start using it that way, it becomes the tool for those things. Then we're no longer in a restrictive diet because we're in a passionate, positive psychology of refueling ourselves. That's really a Zen practice.

Now, here's the hard one that some people will find really challenging, but it's easy, really. I'm going to ask people to do 21 days of a simple 5-minute meditation. The instructions are included, it doesn't have to be formal or anything great, but it gets you back to the ground of quieting the mind in the meditation.

Nothing will replace the potent power and transformative effect of meditation. In this connected, crazy, chaotic, over-stimulus world, we talk about lowering cortisol levels, getting back some freedom, becoming detached from the things that are driving us crazy. We can all get ourselves—I know I certainly can—drive ourselves into a state of despair, hopelessness, anxiety, being completely overwhelmed.

Dean: Yeah, I never get like that...

Shawn: Right... All these states of negative psychology, you really see how transparently self-created they are if you take a 5-or 10-minute meditation break. Get connected to your breath, quiet your mind, stop chasing these rabbits that you're running around, and come out of that and you go, "Wow, man. I was certain the sky was falling in," and all of a sudden, you're standing here going, "Okay, I totally get this. It was just self-created hysteria."

Let's face it. The news, the media, the world as a whole, are really dependent upon us being in this state of hysteria. They'd like to drive it all the time. You hear on the news, a car slides off the road at a

120mph, it's a 20-minute news coverage as if something tragic had happened. Everything is conveyed with a sense of drama, urgency, and crisis. We're all being set into a near-chronic state of crisis, and we expect to function in a highly operative level. It doesn't work.

Getting non-attachment, getting free from the things that are driving us crazy, 5 minutes—it doesn't even take 10 minutes—just practice 5 minutes of breathing meditation in your chair as a given ritual every day for 21 days and see how it works.

Dean: I'm going to try that.

Shawn: You don't have to meditate perfectly or even "right." You just do it. Focus on your breath; breathe air into your belly, allow it to expand, then fall as the air leaves. It's easy, flow and you keep returning your focus to where the air comes and out. The air is coming and leaving. That is all.

There's nothing hard or fancy about it. It's simply quieting the mind. One of the big things is you practice in letting thoughts go, because thoughts come into your mind and they go. You don't grab on. What this does is strengthen your ability to let them go with your eyes open and working. That's all it takes in getting Zen. We'll work on nutritional freedom and mental and emotional freedom through some short meditation.

Very transformative. Now, number 9. Now, we're going back to that yin one. We're going to get game, baby!

Dean: I love that!

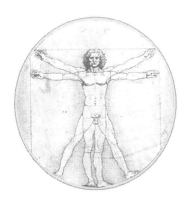

Step 9:

GET GAME

*Competition Fosters Community
and Awakens Your Strength*

Get game is about getting competition. I've noticed this in myself in the last few years. It's the idea that's playing out in CrossFit gyms across the country. A WOD (workout of the day) and a stop watch and you have instant competition—that awakens drive and motivation.

I say competition awakens our soul, our youth, and our spirit. It keeps us honest, focused, and brings out a really masculine energy. Engaging in competitive fire gets you focused and wakes you up. Most people give up competing in anything in their teens or maybe early 20s—other than occasional Frisbee, beer, and golf.

Dean: Isn't it funny when you're in high school and college and in your 20s, everything is a competition. It is all about that.

Shawn: You don't have to run around like the guy who plays too much over-the-top competition and he has to win everything, right?

Dean: Which is just another form of adrenaline-seeking.

Shawn: Yes, exactly! It's as bad as doing none. But as a way to wake yourself up and wake up the game in you, to get your game back, and get your game face on, it's great to engage in some sort of competition, whether it's semi-formal or formal. I've started doing this with some cycling events. I run some crit's (races) or I'll run a time trial. It's amazing what you can do with yourself in an hour if you're under a clock against a hundred other competitors. I'm not trying to win. I don't go, "Oh, I'm going to win this, I bet." It's not to say that I don't try. I did come in third in my first race!

Dean: "I'm just saying that I did come in third..."

Shawn: Yeah, okay. There's that competitive part of me. I've done a little CrossFit, and it's very competitive. CrossFit competitions are actually pretty damn exciting. Impressive and intense. There's something very invigorating and powerful about that.

The same thing happens in the **Body For Life** Challenge, **Bill's *Transformation Challenge***, and it becomes competitive. *Before and after*, you really get your juices flowing when you put some skin in the game.

So, the "**Do This**" just becomes that. It becomes find something competitive. Compete, join a fitness challenge, run a race, ride a timed event, do some CrossFit. Find something in the next 90 days that can engage and activate your competitive energies. **Do one challenge.**

The only thing that doesn't count is you and your buddy betting beers over golf holes. That's not a challenge. But do something competitive that will truly awaken you. Even if you do only one or two a year. A couple of guys, friends of mine, are big mountain climbers. Now, that's a hell of a competition. You've got to be awake the whole time. You're not screwing around.

Dean: Do you think there's some magic about competing against other people?

Shawn: I think for some, there's definitely some magic about competing against other people. For a great example of competition in action, see Strava.com – the online cycling competition. It's huge.

Dean: As part of the man thing?

Shawn: Definitely an awakening thing. The *CrossFit* environment is very tangible. It's hard, but it's very tangible. Nothing like getting beat by women when you're in there. It's like, "Okay..." But I'm not an expert at this yet. I think a really good choice are these body transformation challenges, because they *are* challenges and they're socially conducted, and they're real, especially if you can use a social network to keep tabs on people and to be involved with or train with others. Do you know what I mean? Even having a training partner becomes challenging. You can do it that way.

Dean: Our buddy, Joe Stumpf, just competed in CrossFit and came in 43rd in the world.

Shawn: I know. If anybody hasn't caught the *Kryptonite Report* with Joe Stumpf it's an amazing show. What a brilliant, inspired guy. He's 54, right?

The Kryptonite Report

The **KryptoniteReport.com** is a weekly podcast covering all aspects of living a stronger, fuller more powerful life, inside out.

Dean: When he did it. He's 56 now.

Shawn: He came in 42nd or 43rd in the world in CrossFit in the games. He's got a competitive fire and drive. Part of what woke this up for me was talking to him. Man, who doesn't want to do that? It just makes you want to go. He's got it in spades. By listening to the interview with Joe, you can catch some of that contagious energy. So, that's number 9, ***"Get Game."***

Dean: I love these.

Shawn: You're going to like **Step 10, "Get Big."**

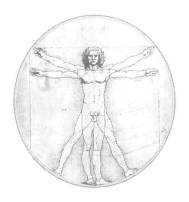

Step 10:

GET BIG

The Truth of Who Your Are is Way Bigger Than The Ego

Get big, man. This is one of the things—and I'm guilty of doing some of these, really struggling—many men develop false, ego-shells in their earlier years, and then they get to 40, and that character strategy is wearing out and wearing on others. Some then stumble into a dose of humility, letting some of the unhealthy parts go, but they're lost without the identity because they had this character strategy that no longer worked. They're waiting for something else to stick to them, or they're wallowing in a lack of healthy ego, or we've been told ego's all bad. There is pathological ego, but there's certainly healthy ego, and healthy ego is part of being a strong force in the world.

I've given ample thought to this topic. When I retired from the sports nutrition company we built, **EAS**, I really thought I had to live as a certain sort of fitness icon. I kept telling myself, I can't ask for this or do that, or I've got to be this thing—this identity. It took me years and probably having children, making a lot of mistakes and a lot of errors to really get that humility where I could just let go and be me. That being me started as letting go of the ego part, which had become an unhealthy aspect of just being nobody.

Dean: Right.

Shawn: Not knowing who to be, you know?

Dean: Right. There's a lot in that, isn't there? It's almost like the Olympic Athlete Syndrome. Their whole life leads up to that one 2-week period at the Olympic Games that's the pinnacle. Then it feels like, "What's my identity afterward?" Especially if they don't win gold.

Shawn: I see that in a lot of players, friends who are ex-NFL players and NBA players. They've been these icons and all of a sudden, they're nobody—relatively. That's not an easy thing to handle. Some of it spews off in some odd ways, including depression. So, I'm not telling people to be nobody. I'm saying, be somebody *else*. But can you choose a healthy BIG you? What I'm talking about is being a **big man** with a small ego by finding your authentic self. You don't have to give up being important to also be a good, healthy, contributing person.

When I listen to *I Love Marketing*, you and Joe have great chemistry, great energy, you've got a great humility. You're humble, but are big characters with big influence. You're interviewing me, you're interviewing Tony Robbins, you're interviewing Tim

Ferriss, Richard Branson... you've got all these people who do all these different things, and you don't treat anyone any differently than anybody else.

Dean: Right. There's something to that.

Shawn: This one's a little tricky, but I think it's about creating a brand that's you but doing it with intention, not just extending your childhood. You had a certain character strategy carried through your teens into your 20s. That character strategy starts to wear and get funky in your 30s. You get into your 40s, and you must recreate your brand.

Who do you want to be?

Dean: It's exciting when you think about it like that—when you think about it, there's an opportunity. When you're saying "*Get Big*," it's getting engaged in a ***bigger future.***

Shawn: Yes. My first "Do This" for "Get Big" is create a 10-year vision. I'm not talking about goals. One of the things that I do really well in *Strength For Life* is separate goals and visions. It's tricky turf because everybody wants to take a vision and turn it into a goal. When they do that, they collapse the opportunity for the vision to be large and inspiring or they set themselves up for failure with their goals.

It's funny (not in a ha-ha way) that we tell our youth to focus on the future, we set vision and plans for our 20's, then some into our 30's and we get to 40 and the focus is not on what we CAN be but what we COULD-A been. That's messed up!

Dean: How do you make that distinction between vision and goals? How do you do that without letting vision fold into goals?

Shawn: I look at goals as tangible markers along the way to get somewhere, so, first of all, my goals are incremental. They're supportive. They're steps along a path to get from here to LA or whatever it is. They're mile markers. So, I want smaller goals that I can achieve and a larger goal that is a bit of a distance away.

But then I look at vision as an inspiring, bright future that lifts me up. I might have a vision of losing 150 pounds. That's not currently a goal. That's the direction that I'm headed towards. My goal is to lose 5 pounds. My goal is to lose 20 pounds. My goal is to ride 150 miles on my bike today. I have goals that are tangible and accessible.

With goals and vision, I like to look to **Newton's law of universal gravitation** that "every mass in the universe attracts every other mass with a force that is *directly proportional to the product of their masses* and **inversely** proportional to the square of the distance between them."

What this means is that sometimes we create these giant massive goals that are too far away to exert any real pull on us. They are attractive but don't' attract us. Or they're too small to attract something even if they are close.

There's a balancing act between a vision being a *giant mass* that has a huge gravitational pull, and goals being small attractors along the way. You have to look at the force—the size and the distance away.

A vision is inspiring, it's as big as I want it to be. My vision for *Full Strength* is simple and clear: *"I believe that the nutrition shake can and should be the most predominant form of fast food in America. And this will make a profound impact on the health and wellness of our country."*

Dean: I think that's a fantastic vision.

Shawn: That's a vision. That's not tomorrow, that's not the next day, and I don't know what the tangible number is when it would be. But that's the direction I'm headed.

Dean: That's the whole vision, I guess. That's the difference. It's not so much you reaching the horizon, but that's the direction you're headed.

Shawn: Yes. We can kill ourselves chasing the horizon because that sets us up for dissatisfaction. Goals give us some satisfaction. So, you want to create a big 10-year vision starting at 40. I'm in my 40s right now. By the time I hit 50, I want to be this *big* person. This *big* person might be *big* in my community, might be *big* in my family. It might be *big* in the life I want to live. It might be that I surf this many days a year. I get to enjoy this much time doing something special. I might be living with Tim Ferriss' *Four Hour Work Week*. I'm making all this contribution, but that vision is the part where we're really remaking our life. We're at this turning point. We're going to intentionally re-craft this next 10 years of our life. It's not going to be an accidental creation of finger painting.

Dean: Right. Exactly.

Shawn: With that is the opportunity to rebrand yourself, to be the big you—big vision, big life, big joy, big love, big mind, big heart. The biggest people or the most authentically big people, not ego driven big people, are the biggest hearts you know. They're not holding on too much. They're not squeezing the joy out of life. They're not in desperation and fear. They're not coming from fear. To be big is coming from abundance, from contribution, from gratitude. We don't get big by strangling life from a position of fear and grasping.

Dean: I'm thinking about what a great word "big" is... "Get Big"—it says all the right things.

Shawn: I think so.

Dean: It really does. It's like you get the idea—it's a visionary word, in a way.

Shawn: I looked at it and said, "Vision is too obvious and too given away." It's just get big, man. Be a big character. Joe's a big character. Dan Kennedy, how big a character is that?

Dean: Right.

Shawn: Love him or hate him, he's Dan.

Dean: Yes, and nobody gets to determine how big you get. Whatever your vision of big is…

Shawn: What's your tolerance? How *big* can you stand to be? How much can you accept and own and not take credit for, but just be good with? I've had a lot of struggle in my own humility around accepting the things that I'm good at. "Oh yeah, I'm okay at that," and finally, I'm like, "You know, I'm pretty damn exceptional at that whole branding thing. I don't know why. I just see things. It's just what it is." And I'm a pretty damn good writer. With all due humility. You've got to accept the things that you do well. That's part of it.

As part of that, going back to getting selfish, I'm pretty good at brand positioning and strategy in the nutrition and supplement business. And I like to help people—it probably feeds my "nice guy" ego. So, for years people have just said, "Let's send Shawn our vision and strategy document on our supplement company because he'll read it and answer everything."

"Let's send him that proposal to buy that company again because I know he'll go through with it." It's because I'm good at it, I enjoy it, I can see market forces, and I can tell you what's going on. But this is changing. I had two "invitations" to share my feedback last month and I sent them an invoice for $50,000 and I said, "That's my day rate. Glad to help."

Dean: Oh, love it.

Shawn: "I'm very happy to help... Here's your invoice." That's not mean; that's just getting selfish. I'm tired of giving what I do away.

Dean: I'm pleased about how all of this has come together. I'm inspired.

Shawn: Well, that's perfect because now we're on to **Step 11: "Get Purpose."**

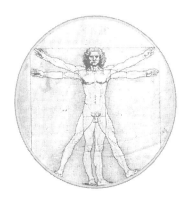

Step 11:

GET PURPOSE

Inspiration Follows Vision
And
Aligns With Purpose

Purpose is a hot word these days. It's a part of awakening as a person, not just men in their mid-life curve. I think purpose is moving toward a stronger community-based society. We've had this pendulum swing toward the rugged individual, so we're moving rapidly back toward a more community centric life, right?

Dean: Yes.

Shawn: We're coming back into community, and purpose is a big thing there. I looked at the whole inspiration because I like to get *inspired*. Inspired is cool. But the reality is, inspiration trumps motivation, but ***inspiration follows vision and aligns with purpose***. If you're on purpose, inspiration is as natural as water flowing down the river.

It's seems we're always seeking to get inspiration, nearly obsessed with motivation but when you get ***on purpose***, it's not about needing the motivation or needing the inspiration because those things come automatically.

I've got a son with food allergies, life-threatening food allergies. I have a ton of purpose around sharing the importance of ***food-allergy-friendly foods*** and *food* safety. I can write stuff on it all day. I can help people all day. I can do anything. I don't need to be inspired by it because I am **on purpose.**

Dean: I love that. When you say inspiration, and when you're on purpose, it's as natural as water flowing downhill, it really becomes that *"Row, row, row your boat gently down the stream."*

Shawn: We're not having to fight upstream to create motivation or inspiration. To be inspired is to breathe in and to breathe out. It's really to be connected to the heart, the meaning, and purpose is really connecting to the heart and the meaning. It's the meaning. We're meaning-making machines. We can't get inspired if we don't have connection to the meaning. You want a great freaking life? **Get on purpose now.** What is purpose other than what Dan Sullivan calls *Unique Ability*? I love Dan. I think I've probably used **Unique Ability** more than any single Sullivan-ation in my life.

Dean: I love that. We've had lots of conversations about it, but the way that he articulates it now in a way that I had never heard it before. He mentioned really concentrating on the *single focused* *activity* that would fascinate and motivate you for the rest of your life. The clues are all right there. It's the things that feel like there's no effort to them.

Shawn: It's what you're doing naturally without any effort. We all have that. The whole key, for me, has always been that it gives you more return than you put into it, so it creates the fuel and energy...

Dean: It's energizing. It's a multiplier.

Shawn: Yes, and one thing I've noticed, being a jack of all trades, is that I'm good at a lot of stuff. I'm really good—I'm better than most people at a good chunk of it.

Dean: At almost everything really.

Shawn: Sure, at a lot of things, and I'm really clear at how some of it drains the crap out of me. If I completely coffee up, I'm good for 3 hours and 12 minutes, and then I'm flat on the floor.

Dean: The 3-hour 12-minute solution.

Shawn: Yeah! Exactly. Boom! And I can't look at it again for 2 days. I can't do another ounce of this; I just can't. It's a desperate state. But with other things... like I can't stop writing. I can be exhausted at 2:00 in the morning and unconscious, then all of a sudden, I'll have this idea and I'll get up and write. I'll do one half of an edit and then people go, *"Wow, where did you pump that one out?"* I'm like, *"I don't know. It just fell out of my hands."*

I didn't really plan it. It's just fell through my head.

Dean: It's what you do!

Shawn: It's what I do. I didn't think I was a writer. I never thought I was a writer. I always— when I started my book, my last one, I hired a writer because I was like, "I can write, but I'm not a writer." Then, I'm like, "Oh, wait. Yeah, I am. Sorry. So, I'm going to have to fire you."

Dean: "Sorry." Yeah, "Forget that."

Shawn: "I'm a much better writer than you..."

Dean: "Thanks for playing."

Shawn: So, get on purpose, man. It's getting inspired and getting connected with your soul's source energy. What is your gift to the world? I mean, especially as guys, if we die with our gift inside us, man, that's not good. That's the worst thing. Guys, give your gift to the world. That's what we're here for.

So, the "Do This" on "Get Purpose" is investigate what makes you tick. I want you to find your *Unique Ability*. Find that thing which you're better at than most everybody, but isn't just something that you exert yourself to do but that actually gives you fuel, that feeds you, that nourishes you, that when you do it, time stops.

Dean: It's like entering a time warp.

Shawn: Exactly, a complete time warp. You lose all track of time. I do that, actually, too often. Ask 3 to 5 people what they see as your gift in you. Ask people. Ask people close to you. It's really interesting to have other people's take and reflection, and often, people will know.

Dean: It's clearer sometimes to other people than it is to you.

Shawn: Yes. They just know that you're exceptional at this. I heard all kinds of things with the Mary Ellen Tribby interview. I'm like, "Man, she's got unique ability at that." You're like, "Wow!" So, it's there. Asking people is a great exercise to take on to help to find your life purpose.

Dean: So, what's your life purpose?

Shawn: I've had this one in my head for probably 5 or 6 years. I think it came out when we were down in Florida. I had it on paper and resonating within me, but I really hadn't taken it out into the world. But my purpose is to help men in the middle of their life live freer, clearer, and stronger lives.

My purpose is to help men in the middle third of life live freer, clearer, and stronger lives.

Dean: When you say that, it really is—it's right in your wheelhouse. It's all the things that you really love.

Shawn: A few years back I redefined the middle-age, into the "middle third" of life because I didn't like the "second half." It's like this; "the first third of life is learning who to screw and how not to get screwed, and the second third of life is making your impact in the world—and wealth—and the third, is giving back." Now, we do all in all phases of life, but I'm really committed to this idea of helping men live fully in this **middle third** of life.

For me, when I turned 40 and started realizing there's a bit of age-related, male discrimination out there. I felt like no marketer, nobody wants you. AARP is the only one that wants you.

Dean: And they show their interest in you too early.

Shawn: Yes. Everything starts going against the 40-year-old man as some trend. How does a guy in his 40s, 50s, gain that foothold, get back on top of life? That, to me, has been my passion. Hence, we're doing the manual, finally.

That bring us to **Step 12: "Get Connected."**

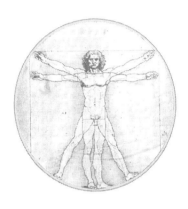

Step 12:

GET CONNECTED

No Man is an Island,
Even if You Own One

I talked about it a minute ago: we're culturally in the phase of our world, our development, and our life, where we're really going back to our community, back to tribes. One of the things I wrote about in *Strength For Life*—what I saw in *Body For Life* transformations—is that you have people who could do it but failed, you have people who changed, and people who truly *Transformed*. The people who transformed, which means they actually changed inside and out—had something in common: they always gave back. They paid their gift forward— always passed on their gift to someone else. They were always in the action of mentoring.

Dean: Wow, that's interesting.

Shawn: So, how do you go from changed to transformed? You get involved, you give back, you get in community, and you share your strength.

Dean: If you think about it, you're creating an environment like in the *Kryptonite Report*. Everything you're doing is creating that community, giving people the opportunity to get connected.

Shawn: Yes, and I appreciate that. That's where I'm going with my whole "Man on Top" (ManonTop.com) conversation, where I really encourage men to *"Get Your Mojo Back!"* –the tag on that community I'm building. I want to get people sharing it forward.

Getting connected—the classic line, "No man is an island"—rugged individualism wears itself the hell out. "I got this one," "I got it," and finally you're like, "Man, can you get that one?"

Dean: Thanks, man. That's great. Super.

Shawn: It's just great. I have had so many experiences in the last few years where I've really worked myself to a position of sacrifice. This is why I teach this stuff because I'm the poster child for a lot of this—self-sacrifice, rugged individualism, "I got this one," "I'm doing it." I've literally had someone go, "Hey, no, no, no. Let me take this," or "I've got this," or "Hey, can I do this for you?" It almost brings tears to my eyes. I'm like, "You want to do this?" "Well, yeah. Yeah." It's a sense of release when someone else is in the game that I can trust to pass this on.

Sometimes I send stuff to people in hopes that they'll say, "Sure, I'll build that." I'm like, "Oh, man." It's really about getting connected, and getting connected is about contribution—whatever your cause is, whatever you're doing in a mentorship, whatever you can do that gets you out and connected.

One of my buddies here in town is the partner in **_Mark Schlereth's Green Chili_**. By the way, if you've never had his green chili, it's unbelievable—the best green chili on Earth. Well, this Wildman, David, goes out on Thanksgiving and slept on the street for 7 days to get 10,000 turkeys for the homeless.

I say, good on you. I'm not volunteering, but that's something. That's a move into community. That's a big move.

One of the things that I want to bring to getting connected, whether it's groups, social communities, golfing communities, cycling communities, mentorship, or $25k groups—anything like that. But there's also an aspect of getting connected at home, which is intimacy and family.

Certainly, I appreciate that I'm not alone in my challenges with intimacy, and I've not exactly been a

4-star general of intimacy. And at this age I get how much that sucks. I regret not opening to it sooner, more courageously. But it always seemed like I was "fine"—and I was, in my head but not my heart.

Dean: "...4-star general!"

Shawn: I'm not exactly a master's level at relationship. I'm just not, but you can't not practice that connection. I mean, I do great with the kids. I've worked my tail off to be better as a partner—more intimate, more connected, and more safe. But, we're out of the John Wayne generation. As much as I'm enamored with *Mad Men*, that isn't exactly the way we get to operate today. While I yearn for a few days of that, ultimately, it would be exhausting. So, there's a part of this intimacy which has to do with an open heart and being present. There's nothing more healing in community than being connected to community and home.

I see a lot of guys that do this really well. They're strength-training, fit, brave warrior types that are also good at intimacy and home life. At the same time, there's a men's movement out there which I think has some threads that are far too feminine. A good balancing aspect of that kind of connection is the book, *The Way of the Superior Man.* (A classic book on The Masculine Journey from David Deida)

Dean: I've heard of it.

Shawn: It's by David Deida. He's probably one of the first movers of the masculine movement (See: *Way of the Superior Man*). I was so offended by the title that it took me a long time to read it, but he has a really good perspective on what the masculine role is and what a man's role is. It's very conducive to good, intimate relationships but it's not the feminine's role.

I like this getting connected, and my "Do This" on these is to just get involved in community. I belong to an entrepreneurs group. I'm in another men's group. Some of the groups can be good and bad, but there are really great rituals, monthly groundings, and places you can go where men have sanctuary— meaning safety, where you can really express yourself safely with men that you know.

I like the man's angle. I think if you have 8 really good men, even in a business group, when you bring in 1 woman, everybody changes their tune and starts talking from a place of ego. It's crazy-making.

You would think it shouldn't happen that way, but it just does.

One of my other "Do This" recommendations is to find a great place to get some ground in the healthy men's movement. Listen to Tripp Lanier's _The New Man_ podcast. Consider The Good Men Project. There are a lot of resources out there. Hell, get into my **_"Man on Top"_** community. I'll get your Stronger, inside out.

Dean: Oh, really? Okay.

Shawn: Tripp has a really well developed podcast. He's a superstar on air. He does a great job with it. He presents a really good, balanced healthy perspective of what **The New Man** is **_"Beyond the Macho Jerk and the New Age Wimp,"_** as he says.

(Find Tripp Lanier at: TheNewManPodcast.com)

Dean: That's so funny.

Shawn: It's a great balance. He just did one with Laird Hamilton, and I love it. Laird's a rock star. I thought it was a great interview about danger, about risk, about fear, about—if you're not afraid of the waves, you're insane.

Dean: Doing those monster waves is crazy.

Shawn: Yes, riding giants. That is certifiable. He was talking about jumping off a 95-foot cliff into the ocean when he was 7 years old.

I'm like, "Dude." He's an adrenaline junkie, but it's a great interview. It's really powerful.

Dean: *The New Man* podcast, okay.

Shawn: So that's getting connected. So, we've come full circle with this.

Dean: I love it.

Shawn: We got real, we got selfish, and we came through all these phases back to connection.

Dean: I love how they build on each other, too. Just the progressive nature of the way they build on each other.

Shawn: Will you read through them again?

Dean: Absolutely. I'll read them. You're thinking about right from the very beginning of "Get Real," then leading right into "Get Selfish." I loved the idea of creating the space for us to get energized. I see already how it's building. When you get real, you're taking this real assessment. Then when you're getting selfish, you're eliminating and creating the space which, by itself, will help us get energized.

Shawn: And if we created energy in advance of the "Get Real" then you're spreading your energy all the wrong places, racing in the wrong direction.

Dean: When we spend this energy, we're going to get strong. I think that right there is shifting this mindset, changing your control from not simply striving to maintain health, but to set the new control we're seeking for strong as the baseline. That's what we're really looking to do.

Shawn: Yes, that's perfect. I love it.

Dean: Then the whole yang of this "Get Gratitude."

Shawn: So, you come back to ground, get into gratitude, the ground of happiness.

Dean: Yes, and "Get Curious."

Shawn: Which is opening, engaging, and that's that beginner's mind.

Dean: I love this: "Get Simple."

Shawn: Yes, now we're clearing. We're making more space. We're eliminating stuff. We're lightening the load of life so that we can soar forward.

Dean: And then, "Get Zen." It's interesting because they may seem very similar when you look at them just on the surface, but "Get Simple" is really about the external stuff, and "Get Zen" is about the internal stuff.

Shawn: That's exactly what it is. You can clear your external world all you want, and it doesn't necessarily clear all your attachments, junks, and filters that are driving you nuts inside.

Dean: Now that you've kind of regrouped them, and set that, now you can "Get Game." It's really building on all of this.

Shawn: Awakening your strength—awakening that natural strength to hunt, compete, and go for it.

Dean: Then, "Get Big." Metaphorically, that's so powerful.

Shawn: Powerful!

Dean: It is! In every way, big is a positive kind of motivating thing.

Shawn: Now, it feels like you're getting this healthy bigness on top of all these parts that you've put together. So, you've got this clearing, you've got this space, you've got all these aspects. Now, you're taking on this new, big identity with this big vision which is clear, aligned, and healthy.

Dean: Then, "Get Purpose."

Shawn: "*Get Purpose*," which is really the ground of inspiration. We want that inspired energy. We want to get aligned with purpose. So, we're getting big, we're getting aligned with our purpose, getting on our unique ability, giving our gift to the world.

Dean: And then, "Get Connected."

Shawn: Which is coming back full circle. Bringing back all our strengths, all our gifts, and really fueling ourselves by sharing our strength.

Dean: Wow. I can imagine being connected with a group of people who are all in alignment with the first 11. Now, you're connected with the community.

Shawn: Yes, and it's a powerful, grounded community because you're all talking the same language, you're all working at the same things. It always reminds me of when *Good to Great* first came out and everybody talked hedgehog, economic engine—the same language. So, we all had the same language, "I want to know how your economic engine is working." This gives us shared community because we have that same language.

Dean: I think this is powerful because you can imagine having this conversation, "Hey, how's your Zen going?"

Shawn: Exactly. You've got a language, a definition, and an action to it. Then I've got the lynchpin action of all, the very last one, the last "get" is actually **Step 13: "Get Going."**

Dean: I like that!

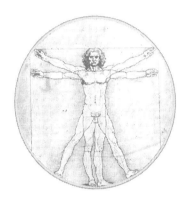

The First and Final Move:

GET GOING

*Life Is Measured in Results
Not Intentions*

Get going now! It's not the best thing to do next week or next year. Take action. Do the small thing every day. I like to say that quantum change is the result of small things repeated daily, not big quantum moves. So, do what? Take a **12-day Reboot**. Clear your life. Take a **90-day Strength for Life** challenge and gauge that.

Here's one of the practices that I've shared with groups in the past, and I'll put in here. It's part of the small things repeated daily. I created this one where I do 9 things in 90 days. What you do is you make a list of "**3 Things to Start Doing**," "**3 Things to Stop Doing**," and "**3 Things to Do More Of**."

3 Starts	3 Stops	3 More of

I like to ask people, "If you did those 9 things in 90 days, what would that be worth to you in your life?" They come up with some number—$1,000 or $1,000,000 dollars, $500—and I give them a silver dollar. "Now, you've got a silver dollar." I tell them to carry it with them every day for the 90 days. "This is your challenge coin, your reminder. This is your anchor that you're making these shifts in your life." At the end of 90 days, you're either going to have a dollar in your pocket or a million dollars' worth of value. Either way you win, right?

Dean: Right, but I mean, really. Compare it.

Shawn: You've got a dollar and a million dollars in value. So, it's get going now with the small things. Take something on and engage. This is probably the foundation for where we need a community to help drive people through these steps. Right now, anybody can begin doing this.

Dean: Yes. This has been inspiring.

Shawn: I'm jacked about it, man. Your question to me, Dean, *"What's the most powerful, life changing thing, that you can do for a guy turning 40?"*

I can offer him some life revitalizing nutrition shakes, help him refocus his life, get some weight off his midsection, and help him feel better about himself, his life, renew his energy, restore hope...But what's the most powerful thing that I can do?

Well, we can do this. These 12 Life Restoring Moves! These matter, these are real.

Dean: Absolutely.

Shawn: These are not huge moves. This isn't a hundred years' worth of work.

Dean: No, it's not.

Shawn: I want these guys to understand, you can read this entire book in 30 minutes. These actions, they're tangible, they're real. It's a guide and a workbook. You've got the space to write your, to do your work. This book, like your life, is full of blank pages. Decide how you want to fill in the years by filling in the pages. Then keep this book with you, live it for the decade.

Dean: That makes it truly the manual.

Shawn: Exactly. I am absolutely certain that the 40's can and should be the best, most enjoyable and powerful decade of a man's life. But that doesn't happen by accident. It happens when you take control, when you live into your truth and vision.

That's what this **OWNERS MANual** is all about. Open your **MANual** and set your course for the best decade of your entire life... *a life at Full Strength!*

Dean: Can you imagine in the world—I mean, not just in their lives—but the impact on the world?

Shawn: It's a completely different trajectory. Instead of hiding your head in the sand, taking the natural order of life, keeping all this stuff you've collected, holding on to all the stories that you've been clinging to, all this stuff and junk you've collected—I mean, the junk in our heads, the junk in our lives, the junk in our hearts. You clear this stuff and say, "Look, I'm going to have another rite of passage here. I'm going to take my 40s and create a new arc, a new uprising, *a new S-curve in life.* I'm going to set a new trajectory, and I'm going to live life as I define it to be for the next 10 years and the rest of my life."

Dean: I just had this vision of what the impact of this message is going to be for people. Thank you for letting me take part in this with you.

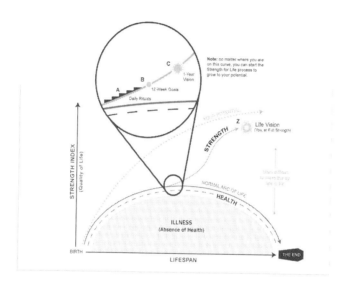

Shawn: Well, thanks for taking the host seat and driving me through, and also for clarifying me to get to the point to do it—this is why you need community. I said it when I came down to visit. I said, "You know, I've been in desperate need to connect outside of my own head and world, and share what I'm doing with other people who can see and reflect." You are able to just look at it—even when I start to get complex or obtuse, you just redirect me back to the simple, you get me back to ground, and I go back to what I know how to do.

Dean: I can't wait to get this out into the world.

Shawn: I know, me either, man. It's been awesome, Dean. I appreciate this. I have to share right now, it is snowing like an absolute banshee here.

Dean: I've got the absolute opposite of that because I turned off the air conditioner so that we wouldn't have any of the background noise, and now I'm sweating.

Shawn: I've got 10 fresh inches of powder right here outside my window. It continues with the yin-yang theme. Dean, this has been a pleasure, and this is a kick-ass special episode of the *Kryptonite Report*.

Dean: I love it. Thanks, Shawn.

Shawn: Alright, man. Thanks, Dean. I'll talk to you soon.

About Dean Jackson

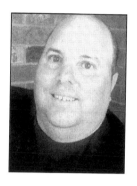

Dean Jackson is one of the world's foremost communicators and influencers. Starting as a real-estate agent in Toronto, Canada, Dean has invested tens of thousands of hours into understanding the motivations, and even more importantly, the resistances of the human condition. As a result, he's amassed a vast wealth of resources, the most important undoubtedly his sphere of influence.

Dean loves helping regular men and women start and grow powerful, rewarding and positive businesses with his "Breakthrough Blueprint" process and can be found weekly sharing his wisdom on the World's Most Popular marketing podcast, *I Love Marketing*. (Yes, find it on iTunes).

Dean is an avid golfer, enjoys a vibrant healthy lifestyle that includes a few episodes of "How it's Made." Dean resides in both Florida and Toronto, depending on the sunshine.

SHAWN PHILLIPS

"The Philosopher of Fit"

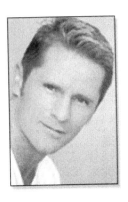

"Your body is strong and vital not because you train; rather you train to celebrate your strength and vitality," says *The Philosopher of Fit,* Shawn Phillips. A deep thinker with a knack for making the complex simple, Shawn's rebelled against the terror of mediocrity since he was a child. Revered for his lean, balanced physique and perfect six-pack abs, Shawn has amassed a lifetime of experience as he enters his third decade as one of the most respected names in the health and fitness world.

Author of the best-selling books, ***ABSolution*** and ***Strength for Life***, as well as thousands of articles on health, fitness, nutrition, mindset, motivation, and more, Shawn brings unique perspective and depth to the questions most fear to ask.

Integrating body, mind and soul, Shawn's *"Zen of Strength"* practice features the techniques of *Focus Intensity Training* (FIT), which blends the intensity of martial arts, the mindfulness of yoga with the muscle of strength training.

Alongside his brother, Bill, Shawn was instrumental in the explosive success of EAS and the *Body-for-LIFE* movement. He pioneered the computerized strength system, ***Powerbuilding***, launched an online supplement knowledge base, Nutros.com and is the founder of the "**lifestyle nutrition**" company, *Full Strength Nutrition*—which helps men live *freer, clearer and stronger in the prime of life.*

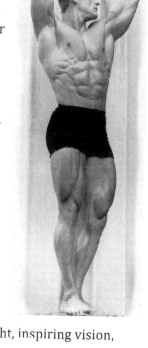

One of the most photographed physiques of a generation, best known for his symmetry and signature abs, Shawn is better known by family, friends and associates for his radical insight, inspiring vision, relentless humor and a passion for helping people live great lives.

143

Find Shawn at:

FullStrength.com The World's Most **Premium Nutrition Shake** (Clinically Proven)

MyStrengthforLIFE.com Shawn Phillips ***Strength-for-LIFE*** the Book site

12DayReBOOT.com **The 1st Move:** Get Your Body & Mind at Full Strength!

StartStrongMonday.com Weekly Wisdom on Strength and Life (Since 2006)

ManonTop.com The Place for Men to Get Your **Mojo Back**

21dayFIT.com The Fastest Fitness Plan on Earth

Kryptonite Report Keeping **You Strong** in a World Robbing You of Strength & Vitality

Neuro-Strength.com Reach Your Peak Strength of **Mind and Body**

Other Creations by Shawn

- ***Strength for LIFE:*** *The Fitness Plan for the Best/Rest of Your Life*

- ***ABSolution:*** *The Practical Solution to Building Your Best ABS*

- ***Full Strength*** *Premium Nutrition for Men*

- ***Red Hot Metabolism :*** *The 7 Immutable Laws of 24-7 Fat Burning*

Made in the USA
Lexington, KY
25 January 2014